ECGs

explained

by

Michael C Colquhoun

BSc, MB BS, MRCP, MRCGP, DRCOG

General Practitioner, Malvern, Worcs and

Clinical Assistant in Cardiology, Hereford County Hospital

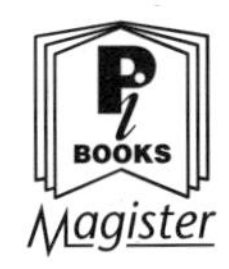

Doral House • 2(b) Manor Road • Beckenham

Kent BR3 5LE

First Published by Publishing Initiatives (Europe) Ltd [Magister] in Great Britain 1997

Reprinted 1998

ISBN 1 873839 29 4

Further copies of 'ECGs Explained' may be obtained from Pi books, a division of Magister. This publication reflects the view and experience of the author, and not necessarily those of Magister.

Printed and bound in Great Britain by S&L Print and Design Ltd.

About the Author

Dr Michael Colquhoun qualified from St Mary's Hospital, London in 1974. After junior hospital posts in London, which included several in cardiology, he became a GP principal in Malvern,Worcestershire. He also holds a post in the cardiology department at Hereford County Hospital. He is currently secretary of the Resuscitation Council (UK).

Author's Acknowledgements

I would like to thank David Pitcher, Consultant Cardiologist, and the cardiac technicians and cardiographers at Hereford County Hospital for many of the recordings illustrated. The remainder were recorded at my surgery, and I am grateful to our practice nurses, Judy Fuller, Mary Jones and Sue Millard, for their help with these. Finally I thank Jim and Ann Silk for their help with producing the illustrations.

Colour slides of any of the diagrams or ECGs illustrated in this book are available directly from the author at:
Court Road Surgery, Malvern, Worcs WR14 3BL
(tel: 01684 573161; fax: 01684 561593).

Electrocardiography was once the province of specialist cardiologists and physicians. Technology has moved on and the specialists have found greater interests in other diagnostic aids; yet the indications for electrocardiography have expanded so that increasing numbers of health-care workers are expected to record and interpret tracings taken in a variety of circumstances. The diagnosis of coronary disease in the community setting is more important now that prevention and treatment have so much to offer, whilst within hospitals, precision in diagnosis has become mandatory for the urgent and effective treatment of heart attacks, rhythm disorders and cardiac arrest. Moreover, electrocardiographic screening is needed for some occupations and has become an integral part of many health checks. But how are the necessary skills in interpretation to be acquired? Training in electrocardiography has increasingly been squeezed from an overcrowded medical syllabus, and its loss is hardly lamented by the teachers whose interests have moved elsewhere. Perhaps much of this very real problem will be met in the future by interpretive algorithms that are already a feature of many electrocardiographs. However, computerised interpretation is not yet reliable enough for most management decisions. It is not widely available either in the community or in emergency settings, and reliance on a provisional report generated automatically offers little boost to work satisfaction. With or without such aids, personal interpretive skills are still needed!

Some knowledge of electrocardiograms is likely to be acquired during early hospital practice, but this is not an area for the occasional expert. Patients have a right to expect competence in the interpretation of investigations: no answer may be better than a misleading one. Those who wish to use electrocardiography have a responsibility to be trained or to train themselves, and in this field - more so than in most - books have a pivotal role. The present text will provide a useful starting point for many.

Dr Colquhoun's book is aimed at general practitioners, nurses, paramedics, and junior hospital doctors and is pitched at a level that is well suited to their day-to-day needs. It gives a simple explanation for the electrophysiological events that are represented as the deflections of the ECG tracing, and it offers useful tips on how to obtain a good quality recording. Appropriately, the changes characteristic of coronary disease receive most emphasis, with other sections on bundle branch block, hypertrophy, tachyarrhythmias, and bradyarrhythmias. Thus, the abnormalities of most importance in general practice and in emergency situations are well covered. The quality of the electrocardiograms is excellent, and the illustrations come with brief clinical histories that add both to the book's educational value and to the interest of readers whose interests will be more practical than academic.

Prof. Douglas Chamberlain

CBE KSG MD Dsc(Hon) FRCP FRCA FESC

Contents

Part C Disorders of Cardiac Rate and Rhythm

Abbreviations

The following abbreviations are used in the text:

AV	atrioventricular
AVNRT	atrioventricular nodal re-entrant tachycardia
AVRT	atrioventricular re-entrant tachycardia
EMD	electromechanical dissociation
LAH	left atrial hypertrophy
LBBB	left bundle branch block
LVH	left ventricular hypertrophy
mm	millimetre
msec	millisecond
mV	millivolt
RAH	right atrial hypertrophy
RBBB	right bundle branch block
RVH	right ventricular hypertrophy
SA	sinoatrial
SVT	supraventricular tachycardia
VAT	ventricular activation time
VT	ventricular tachycardia
WPW	Wolff-Parkinson-White

In this small volume I have attempted to provide an introduction to the subject of electrocardiography. Although the ECG is one of the most commonly performed tests, it differs from most other medical investigations because interpretation of the result is usually the task of the person requesting or performing it. This is particularly the case in emergency situations such as acute infarction or paroxysmal arrhythmia, where the result of the ECG may profoundly influence management. Skill in ECG interpretation requires experience as well as a basic understanding of cardiac electrophysiology. In this book I have explained the electrical events in the myocardium and conducting system that are responsible for the generation of the ECG under normal circumstances, and also provided illustrations of common abnormalities with an explanation of the mechanisms involved. The balance is heavily in favour of the illustrations, which I hope will enable experience in ECG interpretation to be acquired, as well as increasing readers' understanding of the underlying mechanisms involved.

The book is primarily intended for junior hospital doctors and general practitioners, but I hope that it will also be of use to others who use the ECG, especially nurses, operating department assistants and resuscitation training officers.

Michael Colquhoun

May 1997

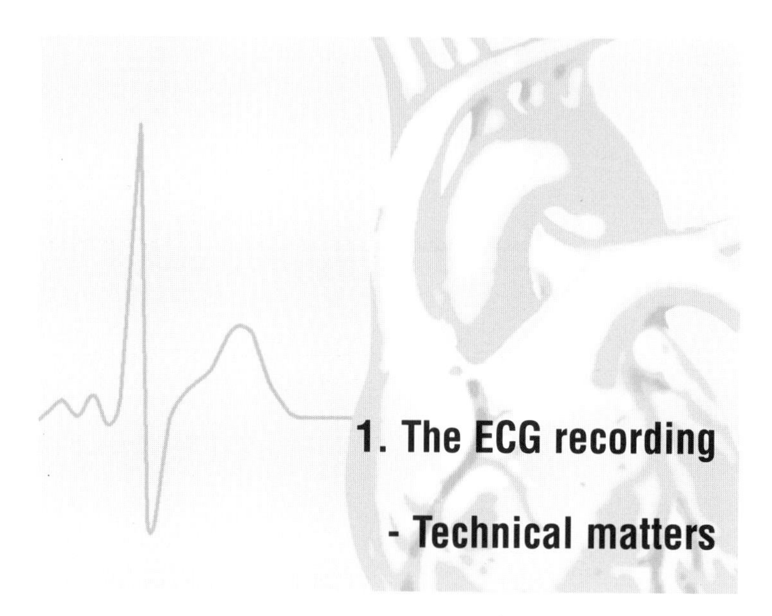

1. The ECG recording - Technical matters

What does the ECG show?

The ECG is a graphic recording of the electrical potentials produced by the myocardium with each heartbeat. Under resting conditions the myocardial cell is polarised, so that a potential of approximately 90 millivolts (mV) exists between the interior of the cell, which is negatively charged, and the exterior. During the process of depolarisation sodium ions enter the cell and the polarity of the cell is briefly reversed so that interior of the cell becomes positively charged with respect to the exterior. This reversal in polarity triggers the actual contraction of the muscle filaments within the cell. The net result is muscle fibre shortening and cardiac contraction.

Each cardiac cycle is initiated by depolarisation of the specialised pacemaker cells of the sinoatrial (SA) node situated in the right atrium. A wavefront of depolarisation spreads outwards from the SA node throughout the atrial muscle to initiate atrial systole. An electrical barrier exists between the atrial and ventricular myocardium, and further spread of depolarisation into the ventricles can only occur through the atrioventricular (AV) node, a specialised group of cells situated on the right of the interatrial septum just below the entrance of the coronary sinus. From the AV node the impulse is conducted to the ventricular myocardium through specialised conducting tissue (the right and left bundle branches and Purkinje fibres).

The electrical signals generated by cardiac depolarisation are conducted throughout the body and may be recorded through ECG electrodes placed on the body surface. The recording obtained from any one combination of electrodes is known as an 'ECG lead'. The earliest ECGs were recorded from two electrodes, each one placed on a different limb and connected to a galvanometer. Electrodes were attached to the right arm, left arm and left leg, and three combinations - leads I, II, and III - were recorded depending on which pair of limbs was selected. Although the original system was chosen largely for convenience, it is still in use today.

Processing of the signal is performed by the electrocardiograph machine to produce the electrocardiogram, which may be displayed on an oscilloscope or liquid crystal screen, or printed onto paper for analysis and storage. By convention, recordings from an electrode recording a positive potential are displayed as an upright deflection on the ECG, while electrodes recording a negative potential display this as a downward deflection. During the cardiac cycle the polarity at any one electrode will vary so that both positive and negative deflections may be recorded. By placing ECG electrodes in different positions relative to the heart, complexes of different configuration may be produced.

ECG recorders

In practice two types of ECG recorder are in common use, the diagnostic ECG and the ECG monitor. The ECG monitor is designed to monitor the cardiac rhythm, and usually has a lower frequency response than a diagnostic ECG. In consequence it will record less detail from the ECG complex, but will be less susceptible to electrical interference or movement artifact. One or two pairs of electrodes are employed to record a limited number of bipolar ECG leads; this is usually adequate for rhythm analysis, but more sophisticated ECG interpretation should not be attempted from such rhythm strips. Cardiac monitors are widely used in coronary and intensive care units where continuous monitoring of the cardiac rhythm is required. Ambulatory (or Holter) monitoring is an extension of the technique used to investigate abnormalities of cardiac rate and rhythm. The ECG signal is recorded for a defined period (often 24 hours) while the patient is ambulant, and is stored either electronically or on magnetic tape for later play-back and analysis.

With the diagnostic ECG 12 leads are recorded, each of which records the ECG from a different perspective; the records obtained from each lead appear different in consequence. The morphology of the ECG complexes themselves provide information about the areas of the myocardium from which they are recorded. Characteristic changes are seen in many conditions, providing diagnostic information and allowing the condition to be monitored by comparison with subsequent recordings. In this regard the ECG has proved particularly valuable in the investigation of myocardial ischaemia and infarction. Some ECG leads may show certain parts of the cardiac cycle prominently and provide additional information; for example lead II and lead V1 usually demonstrate atrial activity well, and are therefore useful for cardiac rhythm analysis. In this book we are primarily concerned with the diagnostic 12-lead electrocardiogram.

In recent years developments in electronics have greatly helped the recording of electrocardiograms. The development of digital recording techniques has simplified the recording process, allowing sophisticated filtering techniques to be applied to eliminate artifact. Digital records are easily processed for storage or computer analysis. The printing techniques used for the ECG obtained by digital recording techniques offer considerable advantages over analogue recorders that utilise ink stylus or hot wire transducers to print the ECG.

Recording the ECG - obtaining a good recording

The changes in electrical potential that occur during the cardiac cycle are relatively small, and sensitive apparatus is required to record them. Unfortunately, there are several other sources of electrical signal detectable on the body surface and these may cause serious interference with the ECG recording. Potentials from skeletal muscle or from nearby mains sources are two common sources of electrical noise, but much can be done to minimise such interference by good recording techniques.

The quality of the signal recorded will be influenced by the contact that the skin makes with the recording electrodes; these must be clean, and electrode gel should be used to ensure good electrical contact with the skin. Hair should be removed where necessary by shaving the skin before attaching the electrode; this is particularly important with the precordial electrodes. The cables connecting the electrodes to the ECG machine must be in good condition, and all other electrical connections must be in good order.

Interference from muscle tremor can be reduced by keeping patients warm and comfortable on a suitable couch that allows them to relax. Explanation and reassurance play an important part in reducing tremor in nervous patients.

Interference from the AC mains can be difficult to avoid, especially where other electrical equipment is in close proximity. The AC mains cables from other equipment should be placed as far as possible from the patient and the cables connecting the patient to the ECG machine. In cases of difficulty other equipment should be switched off if this is possible. Recording ECGs in the patient's home may be fraught with difficulties; substandard wiring and faulty earth connections are often present, and many other appliances that can cause interference may be connected to the same ring main as the ECG machine.

These can often be unplugged while the ECG is recorded, and battery-operated ECG machines may offer some advantages. Most modern ECG recorders incorporate electrical filters that reduce 50 Hz interference from the AC mains, but some loss of detail in the ECG recording results.

The ECG leads

The standard electrocardiogram utilises 10 electrodes - one attached to each of the four limbs, and six placed on the chest wall. Six 'leads' are first recorded using combinations of the electrodes placed on the patient's limbs (leads I, II, III, aVR, aVL and aVF), after which a further six leads (the precordial leads, V1 to V6) are recorded from an electrode placed in six standard positions on the chest wall. There is no logic to the system employed; it evolved in an empirical fashion because certain combinations of ECG electrodes provided favourable electrical signals.

Three standard bipolar limb leads and the three unipolar leads are recorded from three electrodes attached to the limbs. The bipolar leads (leads I, II and III) record the potential difference between a specified pair of electrodes; the original combination derived by Einthoven nearly 100 years ago is still employed.

LIMB ELECTRODES

Lead I Positive electrode to the left arm, negative to the right arm.

Lead II Positive electrode to the left leg, negative to the right arm.

Lead III Positive electrode to the left leg, negative to the left arm.

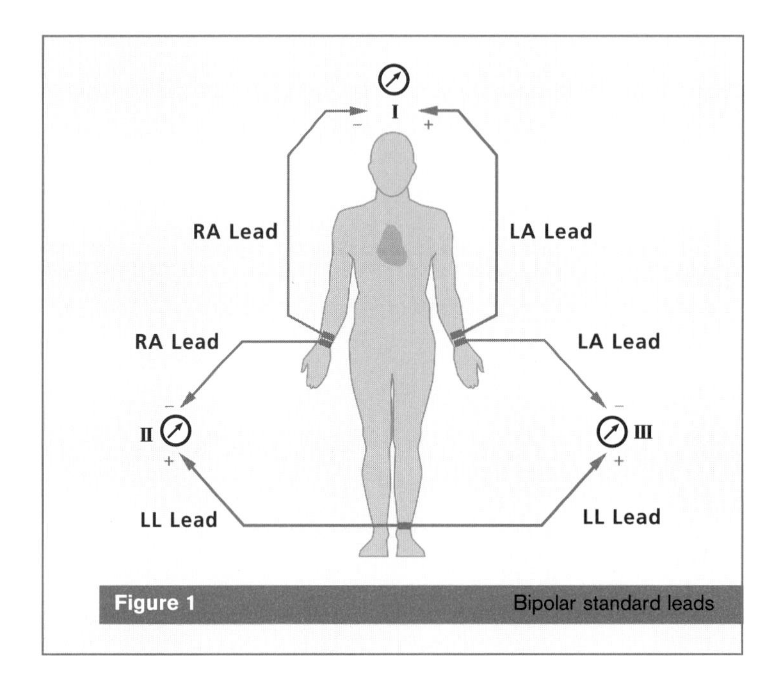

Figure 1 Bipolar standard leads

In practice a fourth electrode is also attached to the right leg, but this is an earth electrode, and does not play an active part in recording the ECG.

The three unipolar extremity leads measure the potential between one 'exploring' electrode attached to a limb with respect to a reference potential derived by joining the other two limb electrodes. The leads, known as VR, VL and VF, record from the right arm, left arm and left leg respectively. The potential difference between the electrode on the limb specified and the average derived by combining the other two electrodes is recorded. In modern equipment the limb connections are slightly modified to obtain an augmented signal and the leads are known as 'augmented' unipolar extremity leads and are designated aVR, aVL and aVF. The electrical connections required to record all ECG leads are made automatically by the ECG machine by turning a selector switch, or by running a programme in the case of automated machines.

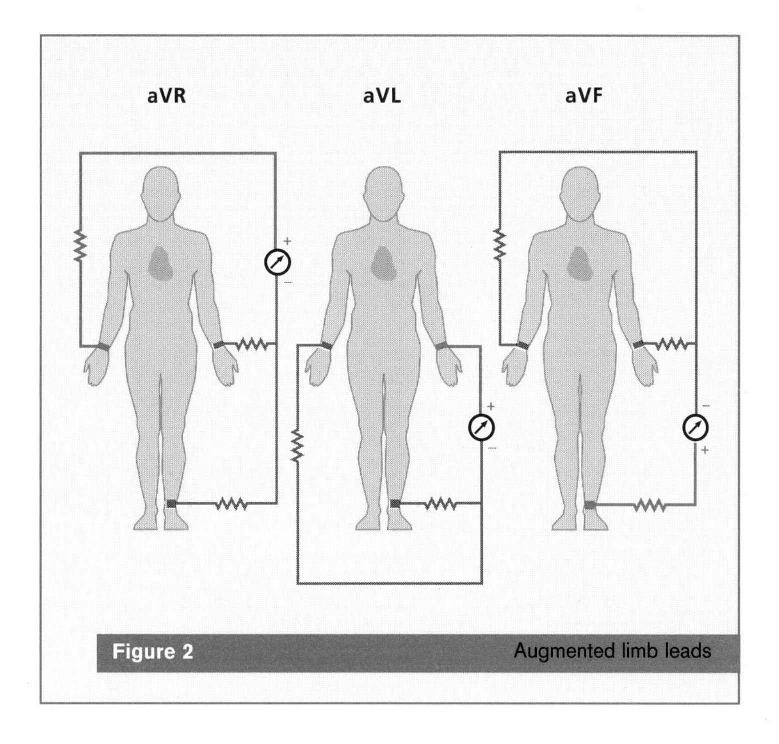

Figure 2 Augmented limb leads

The extremity leads described above record potential changes in the frontal plane and record vertical and lateral electrical forces; they are sometimes known as the frontal plane leads. The precordial leads (V1 to V6), which record horizontal electrical forces, are routinely recorded next. These are also unipolar leads, and record the potential difference between an electrode on the chest wall and the average potential recorded from the three limbs. The chest electrodes must be placed carefully in the defined position if accurate, consistent recordings are to be obtained.

The chest wall electrodes are placed as follows:

CHEST WALL ELECTRODES

V1	Fourth right intercostal space at the sternal margin
V2	Fourth left intercostal space at the sternal margin
V3	Midway between V2 and V4
V4	Fifth left intercostal space in the mid-clavicular line
V5	Left anterior axillary line at the same horizontal level as V4
V6	Left mid-axillary line at the same horizontal level as V4 and V5

By employing a system whereby the position of the electrodes relative to the heart changes with each ECG lead recorded, the 12-lead ECG contains 12 different records of cardiac electrical activity. In other words, each of the individual leads records the ECG from a slightly different perspective.

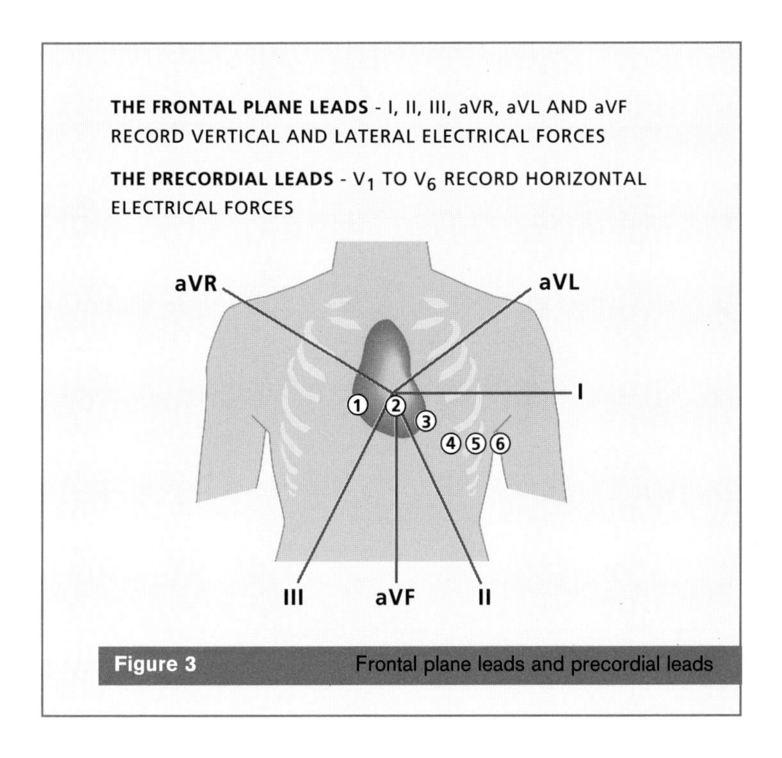

Figure 3 Frontal plane leads and precordial leads

The relative positions from which the various ECG leads look at the heart are shown in *Figures 3 and 4*. The unipolar extremity leads can be considered to record from the right shoulder (aVR), the left shoulder (aVL) and from directly below the heart (aVF). Lead I records from the left side of the heart from a point inferior to the left arm lead (aVL). Lead II records from a point to the left of the foot lead (aVF) while lead III records from a point to the right of this lead.

The distribution of these leads around the heart is uneven, being biassed towards the lateral and inferior surfaces of the heart. Leads I and aVL record from the anterolateral surface of the heart, while leads II, III, and aVF record from the inferior surface. Lead aVR looks downwards into the heart and the recording obtained resembles an intracavitary recording.

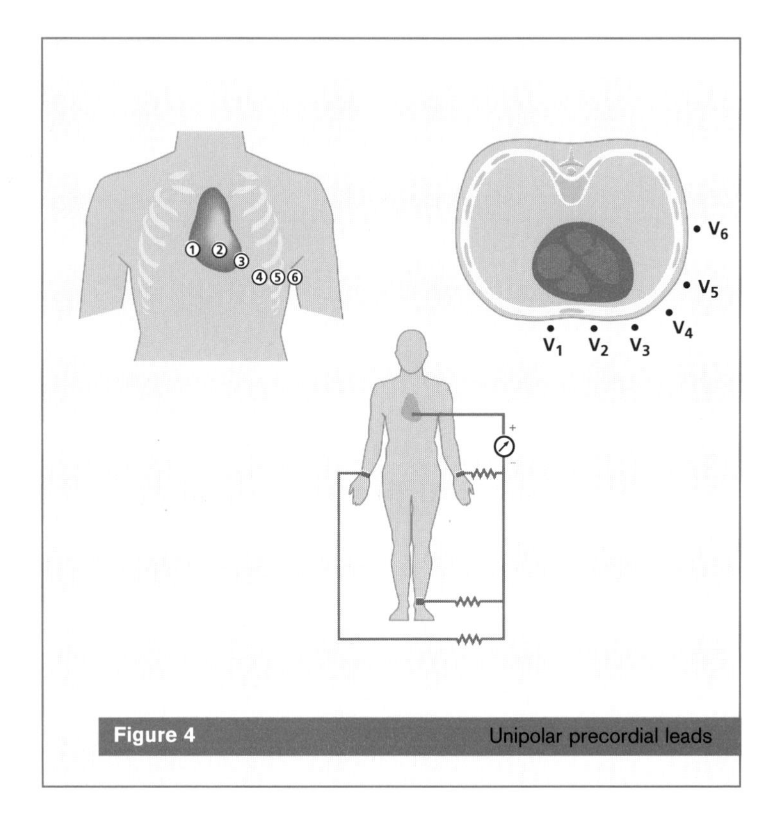

Figure 4 Unipolar precordial leads

The precordial leads record directly over the myocardium, and give information about a localised area. Leads V1 and V2 lie above the free wall of the right ventricle. V3 lies over the interventricular septum. Lead V4 records from near the septum and from the region of the apex of the left ventricle. The final precordial leads, V5 and V6, lie over the free wall of the left ventricle. In fact other

V leads can be recorded by placing the chest wall electrode more posteriorly in the axilla and on the posterior chest wall. These are occasionally employed to obtain information from the lateral and posterior surface of the left ventricle.

The ECG recording

The ECG is recorded on graph paper calibrated in millimetres (mm). To facilitate the inspection of traces, every fifth line (on both the horizontal and vertical axis) is accentuated by bolder printing. A standard recording speed of 25 mm per second is used in the UK so that every millimetre of graph paper on the horizontal axis represents 40 milliseconds (msec). The bolder lines on the horizontal axis therefore represent 200 milliseconds.

The amplitude of the fluctuations in electrical potential recorded by the ECG is displayed on the vertical axis. A standard calibration of one millivolt (mV) per centimetre is employed, and this calibration should be recorded on the ECG at the start and end of the record. Manual machines usually have a mechanism for printing the standard 1 mV calibration signal; this is done routinely with automated machines. The size of the deflections in the vertical plane, especially of the QRS complexes, have diagnostic implications, and accurate recording techniques are essential if reliable results are to be obtained. Although it is possible to describe the deflections on the vertical axis in voltage terms (i.e. 1 mm equals 100 microvolts etc.), the height or depth of the deflections is usually described in millimetres measured directly from the ECG paper.

ECGs were traditionally printed as a continuous strip with each ECG lead recorded separately and printed in succession in the order already described. Modern three-channel machines print the ECG on one side of A4 graph paper. In the illustrations in this book three leads are recorded simultaneously for approximately 2.5 seconds, after which the machine switches automatically to the next three leads. Leads I, II and III are recorded in the first time period, leads aVR, aVL and aVF in the second, leads V1, V2, and V3 in the third period followed by V4, V5 and V6. The three leads recorded in each time period are usually printed vertically above each other. The 10 seconds of cardiac activity recorded in the four time periods are printed continuously on the long axis of an A4 sheet of paper. A 10-second rhythm strip is also printed at the foot of the page underneath the 12-lead ECG. Some machines offer a choice of alternative report formats, but this is the one chosen for the ECGs illustrated in this book. Most three-channel ECG machines also incorporate a control to enable the continuous recording of any one of the three-lead combinations for as long as the operator requires; this is particularly valuable in the investigation of arrhythmias and their response to treatment.

It is essential that documentation of the patient's details is included on the recording. The very minimum must be the name of the patient, with the date and time at which the ECG was recorded. This information should be entered on the ECG immediately the record has been taken, either at the start or end of the recording; do not write on the paper that contains the actual ECG trace.

If the ECG recorder does not label the individual ECG leads automatically, it is well worth doing this as soon as the record is complete. The task can become very much more difficult later, especially when a lead has been recorded more than once because of technical problems. Some modern ECG recorders enable the entry of considerable amounts of patient information through a keyboard, and this is subsequently printed on the recording.

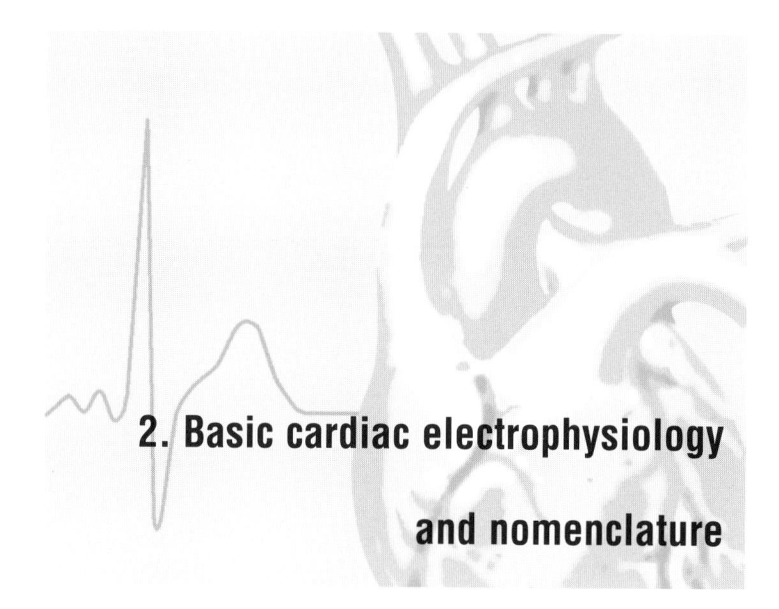

2. Basic cardiac electrophysiology and nomenclature

Electrical activation of the heart

An understanding of the sequence of cardiac depolarisation is required to appreciate how the ECG is produced. The subsequent application of these basic principles will greatly facilitate the systematic interpretation of the ECG.

Contraction of cardiac muscle fibres occurs after the cell membrane has become depolarised; it is the process of depolarisation (and subsequent repolarisation to restore the cell to its resting state) that is recorded by the ECG. Under normal circumstances the cardiac muscle cells (and the specialised conducting tissue of the heart) are polarised; a potential difference of approximately 90 mV exists between the interior of the cell (which is positively charged) and the extracellular space. Reversal of this electrical charge (the process of depolarisation) leads to calcium entry and contraction of myocardial cells.

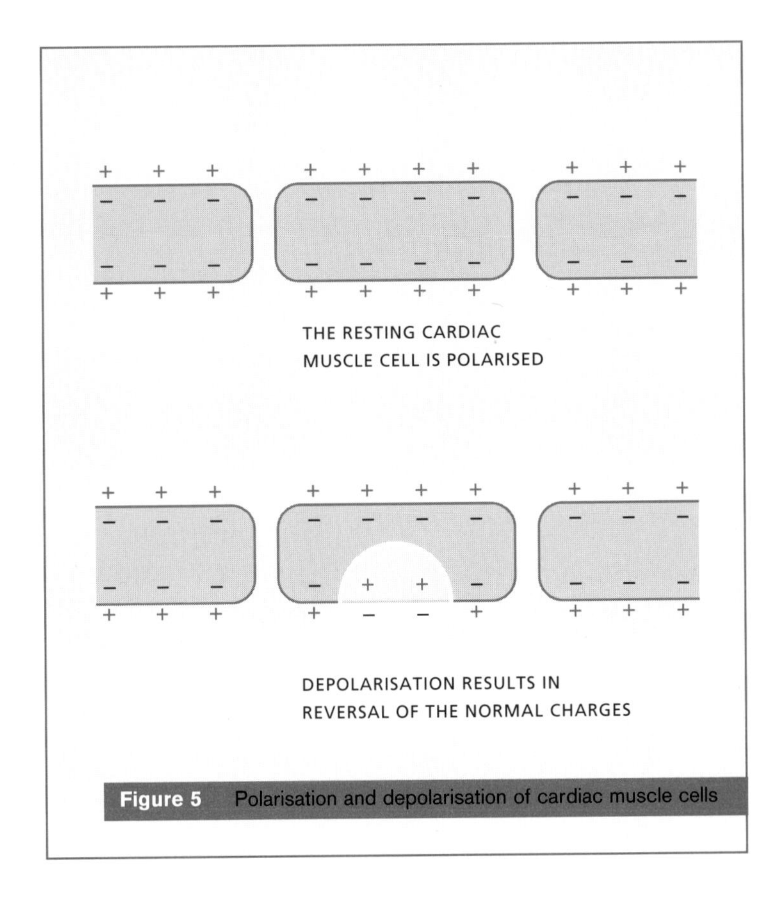

Figure 5 Polarisation and depolarisation of cardiac muscle cells

Under normal circumstances depolarisation is initiated from a group of specialised pacemaker cells (the sinoatrial node) situated in the right atrium. Depolarisation spreads from the SA node into the surrounding atrial myocardium and is propagated throughout both the atria to produce atrial systole. Depolarisation of the atria is recorded on the ECG as a deflection known by convention as a P wave.

Further spread of depolarisation to ventricular myocardium occurs through specialised conducting tissues - the atrioventricular (AV) node and His-Purkinje system. The AV node and bundle of His (sometimes called the AV junction) are situated in the lower part of the right atrium just above the interventricular septum. Depolarisation spreads distally from the AV junction through two specialised bundles of conducting tissue, the right and left bundle branches, which in turn divide into a network of Purkinje fibres that supply the right and left ventricle respectively.

Depolarisation of the ventricles produces a deflection on the ECG recording known as the QRS complex; ventricular contraction follows.

Repolarisation of the ventricular myocardium (the process by which the resting potential of the muscle is restored) occurs after a short delay (the ST segment) and is represented on the ECG as the T wave. Atrial depolarisation may sometimes be seen on the ECG after the P wave (when it is known as a Ta wave), but is a small deflection and often obscured in the early part of the QRS complex.

Nomenclature, definitions and measurements

The PQRSTU nomenclature of the ECG waveforms originally described by Einthoven almost 100 years ago is still universally employed. Below are the most important terms used in ECG interpretation.

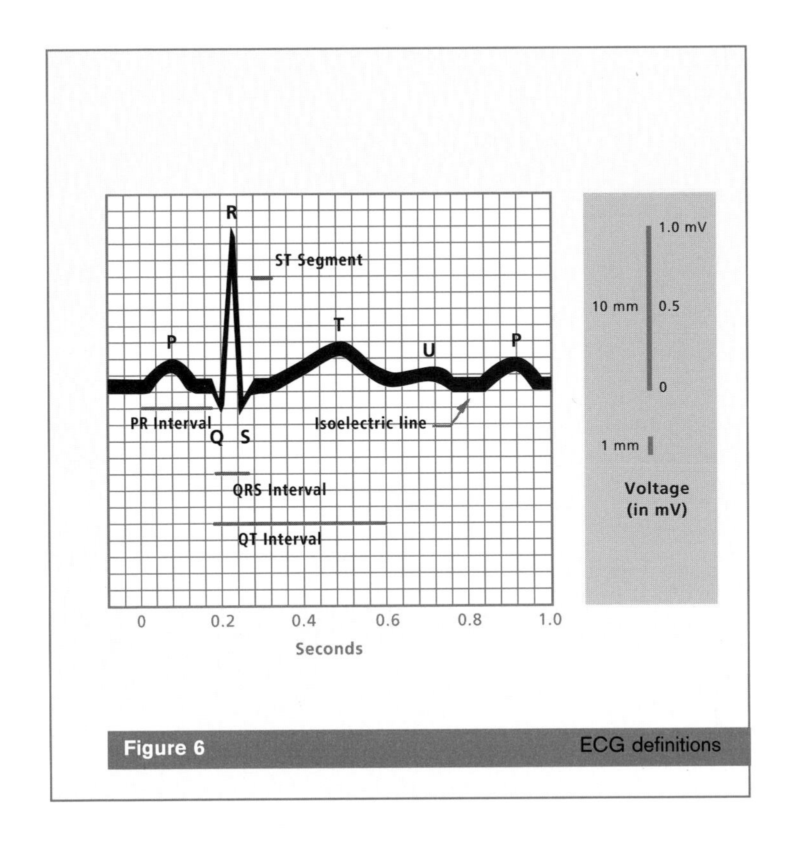

Figure 6 ECG definitions

NORMAL ECG COMPLEXES

P wave The deflection produced by atrial depolarisation. It is the first deflection of the ECG in the cardiac cycle. It is normally well seen in leads II and V1, and normally less than 3 mm (300 microvolts) in amplitude, and less than 3 mm (120 msec) in duration.

QRS complex This represents the spread of depolarisation throughout the ventricular myocardium and is usually the largest deflection of the ECG. The complexes may start with either a negative or a positive deflection, and may have two or more recognisable deflections within them. By convention large deflections (greater than 500 microvolts or 5 mm of ECG paper) are designated with capital letters, while lower case letters are used for smaller deflections.

The Q (q) wave is the first negative deflection arising from ventricular activation, and precedes the first positive deflection, the R (r) wave. A complex that is entirely negative is known as a QS wave.

The R (r) wave is the first positive wave of the QRS complex; it may not necessarily be preceded by a Q (q) wave. Any second positive deflection in the QRS complex is known as an R' (r') wave and will follow an S wave.

The S (s) wave is the first negative deflection to follow a positive deflection (an R or r wave). A negative deflection following an R' wave is termed an S' wave.

T wave The deflection produced by ventricular repolarisation.

U wave A deflection following the T wave and preceding the next P wave. The origin of the U wave is poorly understood; repolarisation of the conducting tissue has been proposed as its source.

ECG INTERVALS

PR interval This is the time between the first deflection of the P wave and the first deflection of the QRS complex.In many cases this will in fact be the PQ interval, but the term PR interval is widely used. It represents the time interval between the onset of atrial depolarisation and the onset of ventricular depolarisation. This in turn is made up of the time required for atrial depolarisation plus the delay to conduction that occurs in the AV node. The normal range is 120-210 msec. The interval is short when ventricular activation occurs more rapidly than normal (for example when the AV node is bypassed by abnormal conducting tissue) and is prolonged when AV conduction is delayed.

QRS interval (or duration) This is a measurement of the total time occupied by ventricular depolarisation. It is measured from the first deflection of the QRS complex (whether this is a Q wave or an R wave) to the end of the QRS complex (whether this be the end of a positive or negative wave). The upper limit of normal is 100 msec (2.5 mm of ECG paper).

QT interval This is measured from the start of the QRS complex to the end of the T wave. The duration varies with heart rate, and formulae that correct for changes in heart rate (the Q-Tc) are available. The Q-Tc should not exceed 420 msec.

ST interval (segment) This is the part of the tracing between the end of the QRS complex (known as the J point) and the onset of the T wave. The actual duration has little practical significance, and is difficult to measure consistently. More important is whether the segment is elevated or depressed in comparison with the baseline between the termination of the T wave and the beginning of the P wave.

R-R interval This is the distance between the same point on two successive R waves. When the rhythm is regular, the time between two successive R waves divided into 60 gives the heart (QRS) rate. When the rhythm is irregular, the number of R waves in a specified time period can be used to calculate the QRS rate.

An alternative method of calculating heart rate is to divide the R-R interval measured in millimetres into 1500.

P-P interval This is the distance between the same point of two consecutive P waves. In normal sinus rhythm this will be the same as the R-R interval.

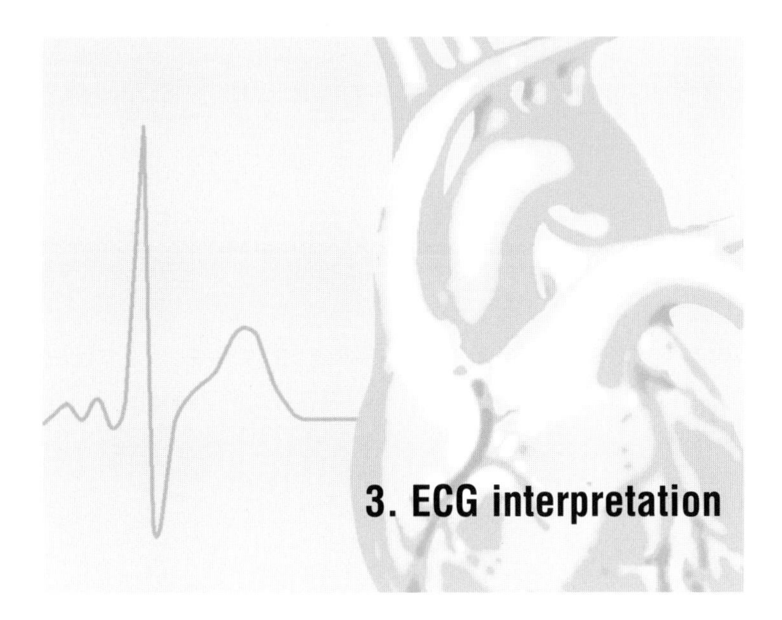

3. ECG interpretation

The ECG records the changes in electrical potential that result from depolarisation and repolarisation of the myocardium. Atrial and ventricular depolarisation are recorded separately, and the sequence of electrical activation of the heart determines the cardiac rhythm. One of the major applications of electrocardiography is in the analysis and treatment of disorders of cardiac rhythm and conduction.

The shape and size (i.e. the morphology) of the deflections of the electrocardiogram provide further information about the cardiac chambers from which the ECG is derived. The presence of myocardial ischaemia or infarction can be diagnosed by certain characteristic morphological changes in the QRS complexes, ST segments and T waves. The presence of chamber hypertrophy can be deduced when the voltages of the deflections derived from the chamber are increased. This is particularly the case in left ventricular hypertrophy where the voltages of the QRS complexes are increased.

A systematic approach to interpreting the ECG should be adopted routinely, and with experience will become second nature. By being thorough and methodical, the information available from each ECG will be maximised and mistakes through overlooking something will be avoided. Several schemes of ECG interpretation have been proposed, many of which differ in detail only. The following is suggested as a framework to work within. It is not a rigid protocol; in many cases the interpretation will be determined by the clinical circumstances. In a collapsed patient with tachycardia, the analysis of cardiac rhythm will be the first consideration. In a patient with chest pain, analysis of the QRS complexes, ST segments and T waves (to assess evidence of ischaemia or infarction) will predominate. Whatever the reason for performing the ECG, however, the interpretation should nevertheless be comprehensive.

Patient documentation

Check this every time you are asked to interpret an ECG; it is embarrassing as well as potentially dangerous to apply the findings of an ECG to the management of the wrong patient. When recording the ECG yourself always document the patient's identity and the date and time of the recording.

Clinical details

Ideally the interpretation of the ECG is undertaken by someone aware of the clinical context in which the ECG was recorded; this is often the person managing the patient. Many important ECG changes (particularly of the ST segment and T wave) can only be interpreted in the light of the clinical context in which the ECG was recorded. Associated information about blood pressure, drug treatments and coexistent medical conditions has major relevance to ECG interpretation, and routine ECG reports provided without this information are usually of limited value.

Technical quality

A quick scan of the ECG is usually sufficient to detect major problems caused by interference or inadequate recording technique. The calibration signal is also conveniently checked at this stage.

Assess the rhythm

The cardiac rhythm present on the ECG should be defined at an early stage. The analysis of cardiac rhythm and conduction disturbance is the subject of Part C of this book.

Assess the morphology

The QRS complexes are usually examined first. The principal morphological features of importance are the presence of pathological Q waves which may indicate previous infarction, and the amplitude of the QRS deflections. Increased QRS voltages may signify ventricular hypertrophy, while loss of R waves in leads where they would be expected to be present may indicate lost myocardium, usually the result of infarction. The QRS complex width should be examined routinely; prolongation has important implications for the interpretation of morphological abnormalities as well as rhythm disturbance. It does not matter whether the limb leads or the precordial leads are examined first; it is a personal decision.

Examination of the ST segment and T wave is inextricably linked with analysis of the QRS complex, and is therefore best performed at this stage.

The P waves will already have been assessed during the analysis of cardiac rhythm, and in many cases the principal value of the P (or other electrocardiographic evidence of atrial activity) is in the analysis of rhythm disturbance. When sinus rhythm is present, however, morphological abnormalities of the P waves do have additional significance, for example in the diagnosis of atrial hypertrophy. The PR interval should be assessed in all ECGs where P waves are present.

The interpretation of many of the more common morphological abnormalities encountered is illustrated in the examples contained in the following chapters.

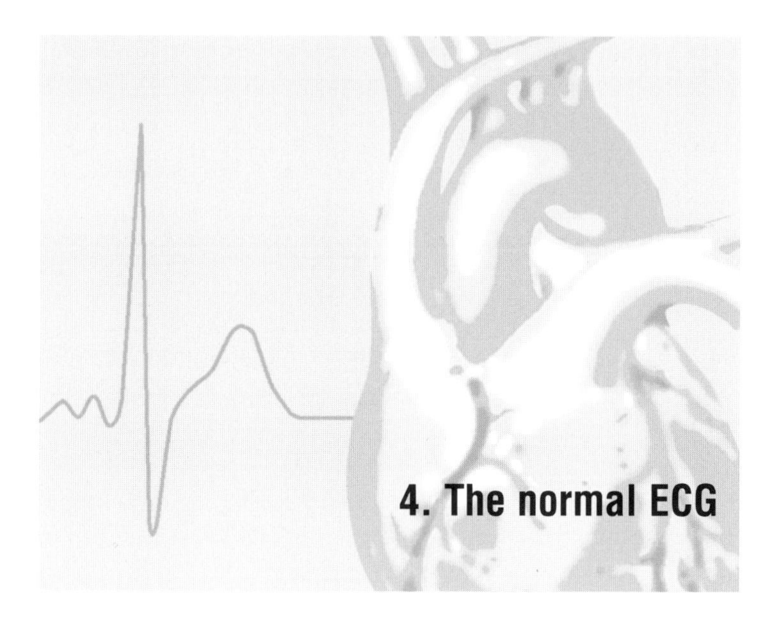

4. The normal ECG

In this section (Chapters 4 to 7) some of the normal ECG features and common morphological ECG abnormalities encountered in clinical practice are illustrated. The patient in whom the ECG was recorded is briefly described and I hope this places the ECG findings into context and helps the reader appreciate the value of the ECG in the management of patients. At the same time I also hope to illustrate the limitations of the ECG, which is often not a very sensitive instrument in establishing a diagnosis. Neither are many of the ECG changes encountered very specific for a particular condition; this is well illustrated by the abnormalities that occur in the ST segment and T wave.

It must also be appreciated that the ECG does not provide an aetiological diagnosis; for example the ECG may show strong evidence of left ventricular hypertrophy, but the cause of this (which might be hypertension, hypertrophic cardiomyopathy, valvular disease or a combination of conditions) can only be established by correlating the ECG changes with the clinical findings in the individual patient.

Case 1: ECG recorded for insurance purposes in a 30-year-old man

The rhythm is sinus at a rate of 57 per minute; sinus bradycardia is present.

Limb leads: The record is different in each of the six leads because of their differing orientation to the heart. Note how all the limb leads except aVR and aVL record a predominantly positive deflection. The largest positive QRS deflection is recorded in lead II indicating that the main electrical vector resulting from left ventricular depolarisation is directed towards that lead. Lead aVR records from the right shoulder and looks into the cavity of the heart. All the electrical forces are directed away from this electrode which therefore records negative P, QRS and T deflections. Recording from a point almost diagonally opposite lead II, it is interesting to note that the ECG recorded by aVR is an inverted version of that recorded in lead II.

Precordial leads: There is an R wave in all leads, and the amplitude of this increases progressively from V1 to V4 after which it declines. An S wave is present in V1 and increases progressively to lead V3 after which it declines, although it is still present in V6. A small negative Q wave is seen as the initial deflection of the QRS complex in V5 and V6. This is less than 40 msec in duration and less than 25% of the height of the following R wave, and is therefore a non-pathological Q wave. The magnitude of the QRS deflections is within normal limits (see later), and the QRS duration is less than 100 msec and is therefore normal. The ST segments are isoelectric.

The T wave is upright in all leads except aVR (where inversion is normal for reasons that we have already seen), and in lead V1 (where inversion is also normal). The T wave may also be normally inverted in lead V2 if it is inverted in V1, but it is upright in this case.

ECG 1

Recorded for insurance purposes in a 30-year-old man

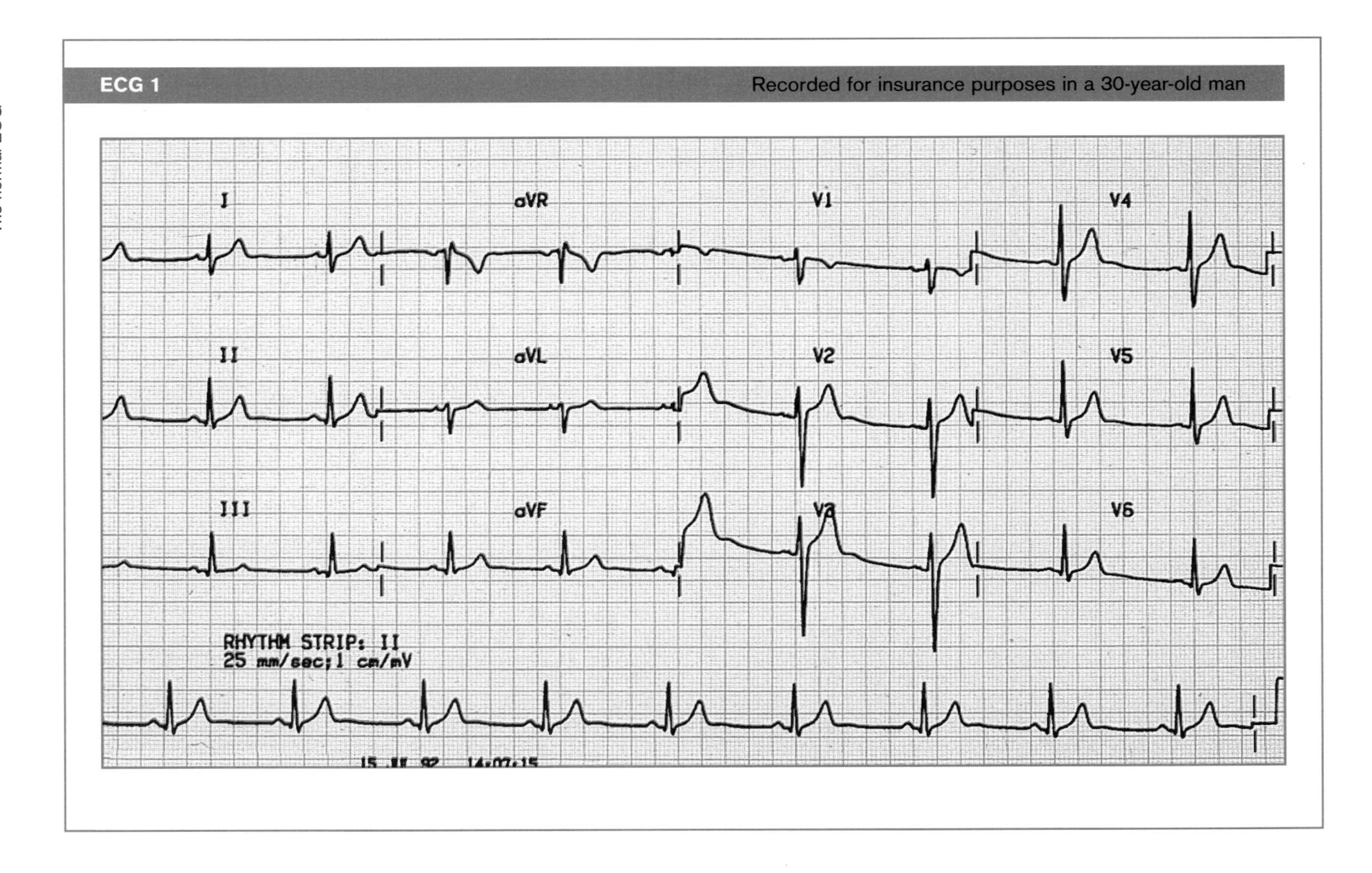

Case 2: ECG recorded from a 32-year-old cardiac technician to test a new ECG machine

Sinus rhythm at a rate of 75 per minute is present.

Limb leads: As in the previous example the greatest positive deflection is recorded in lead II. Lead III records only a very small QRS complex implying that the net electrical vector resulting from ventricular depolarisation is directed at right angles to the electrode. No electrical forces directed towards or away from the lead III electrode - which would cause positive or negative deflections respectively - are recorded.

Precordial leads: Initial R waves are seen in the right-sided precordial leads V1 and V2, and the height of the R wave increases progressively as the electrodes progress to the left across the chest. Small q waves are recorded in the left-sided leads V5 and V6. Deep S waves are seen in V1 and these become progressively smaller as the recording progresses across the chest - it is just visible in V6 as a small negative deflection after the R wave.

The small R waves in the right-sided leads and the small Q waves in the left-sided leads result predominantly from depolarisation of the interventricular septum (which is depolarised from the left bundle branch, i.e. from left to right). A lead on the right of the chest (e.g. V1 or V2) therefore records a positive deflection while one on the left of the chest (e.g. V5 or V6) records a negative one. Part of the R wave in right-sided leads also results from early activation of the anteroseptal area of the right ventricle. This is also directed towards the leads and so further increases the height of the R wave in these leads.

The deep S waves in the right-sided leads and the tall R waves in the left-sided leads represent ventricular depolarisation. The muscle mass of the left ventricle far exceeds that of the right, and the electrical forces generated by the left ventricle are far greater than those by the right. Depolarisation of the left ventricle is therefore responsible for the majority of these deflections. A negative S wave is recorded in V1, V2 and V3 because the main electrical forces resulting from ventricular depolarisation are directed towards the left, away from these electrodes. Positive deflections are recorded from electrodes placed further to the left that overlie the left ventricle - in this case leads V4, V5 and V6.

ECG 2

Recorded from a 32-year-old cardiac technician to test a new ECG machine

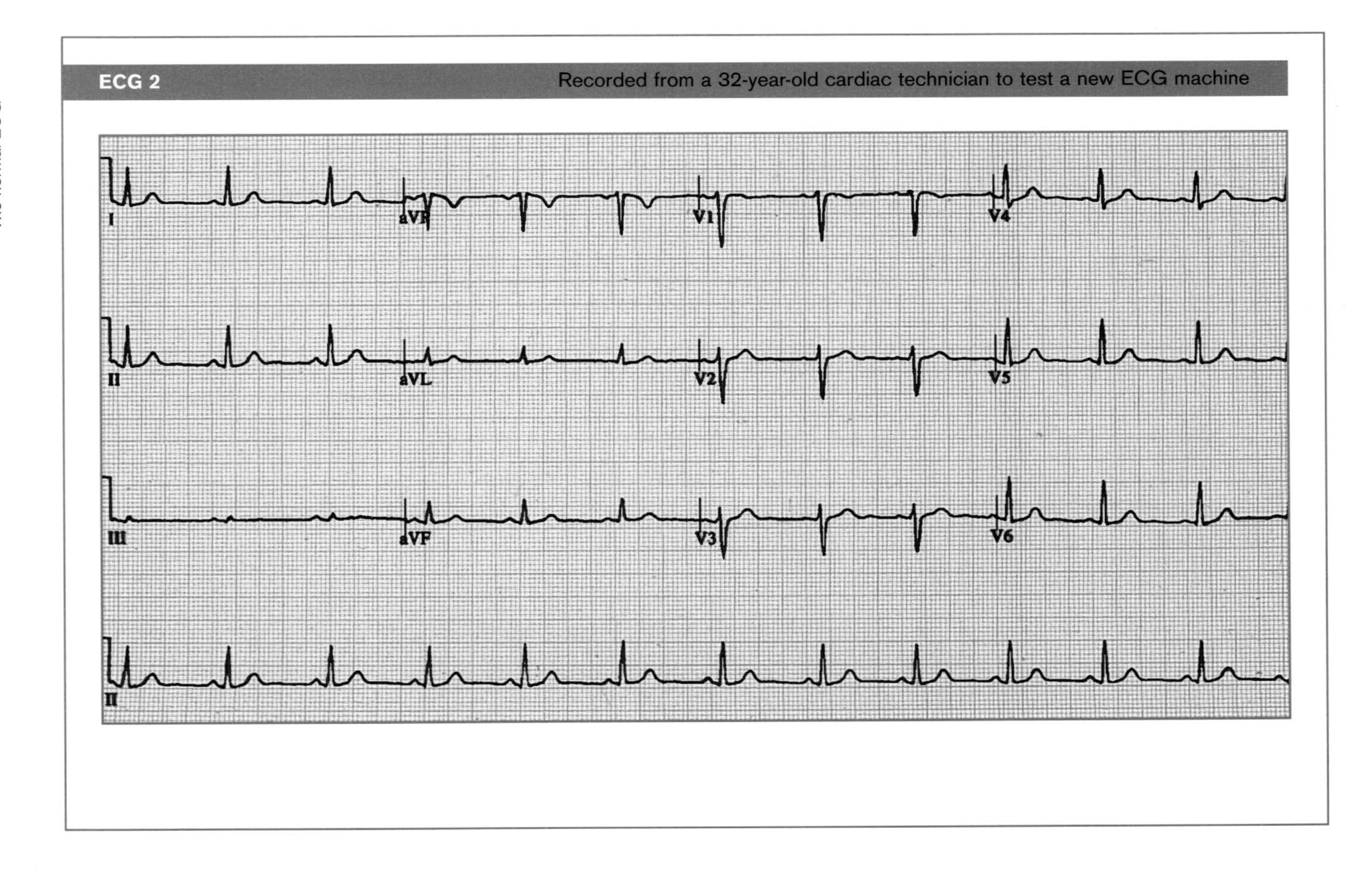

Case 3: ECG recorded in a 61-year-old woman who complained of palpitation

Sinus rhythm at a rate of 75 per minute is present.

Limb leads: The greatest positive QRS deflection is recorded in lead I. This occurs because the mean electrical forces generated during ventricular depolarisation are directed towards that lead. This vector of this force is directed away from lead III, which therefore records a negative Q wave. This is not a pathological Q wave and should not be interpreted as an indication of previous inferior infarction. In the case of inferior infarction, pathological Q waves are usually seen in leads II and aVF as well as in lead III. The isolated Q wave in lead III demonstrated in this case often fluctuates with respiration, and may even disappear completely as the position of the heart changes during deep inspiration.

Precordial leads: In the normal cardiac position V1, V2 and V3 overlay the right ventricle and leads V4, V5 and V6 overlay the left ventricle. The direction of depolarisation of the interventricular septum is from left to right and therefore towards leads V1, V2 and V3, which record an initial positive r wave. Left ventricular depolarisation which then follows is directed from right to left and is responsible for the deep S waves seen in these leads.

Septal depolarisation occuring in a direction away from leads V4, V5 and V6 is responsible for an initial negative q wave in these leads. In practice, this may be so small as to be difficult to see. Left ventricular depolarisation is subsequently directed towards these leads and is responsible for the dominant R waves recorded in these leads. The region where the deflection changes from a dominantly negative S wave to a dominant R wave is known as the transition zone, and in this case occurs between leads V3 and V4. It usually corresponds to the site of the interventricular septum.

ECG 3

Recorded in a 61-year-old woman who complained of palpitation

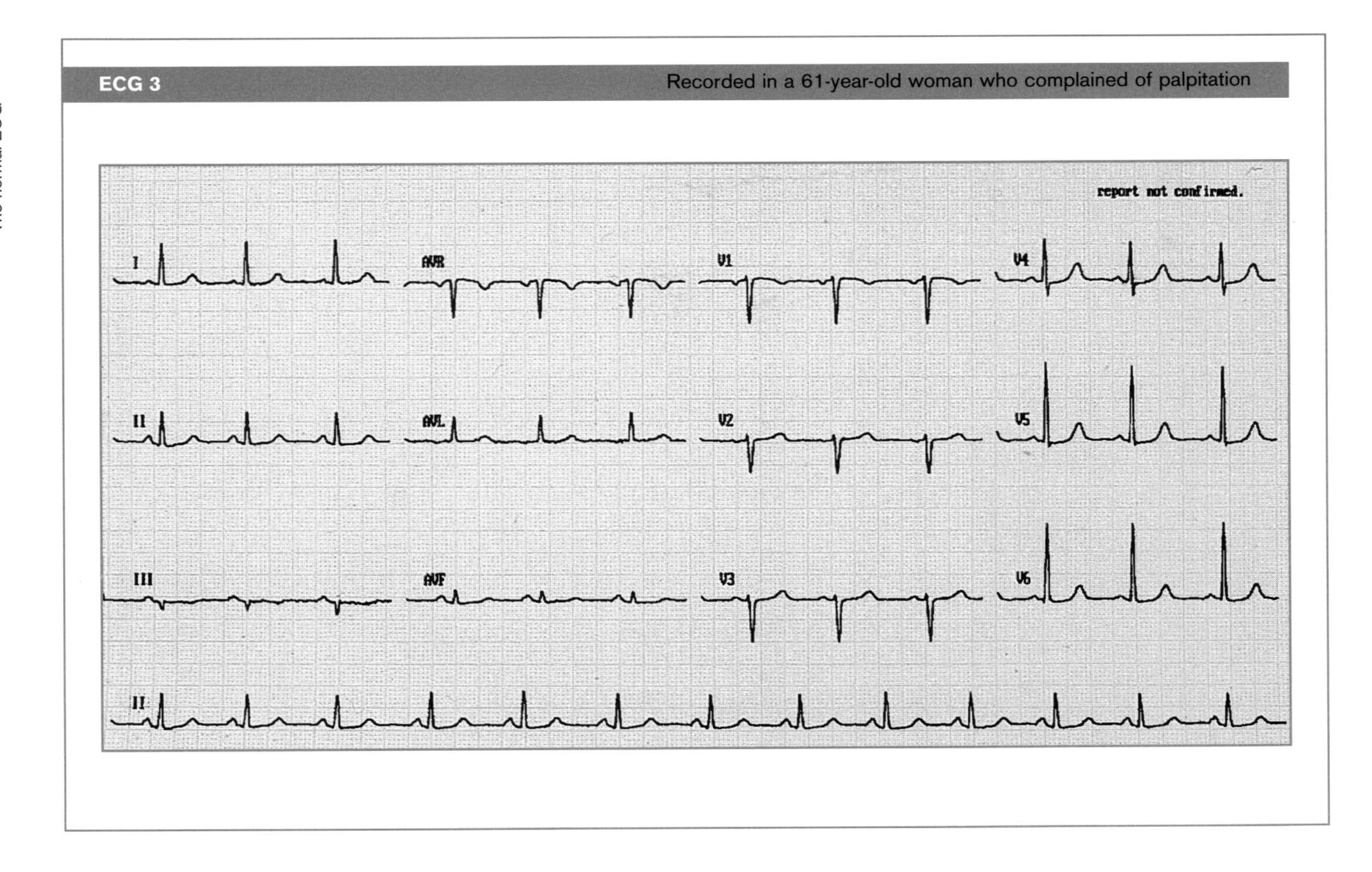

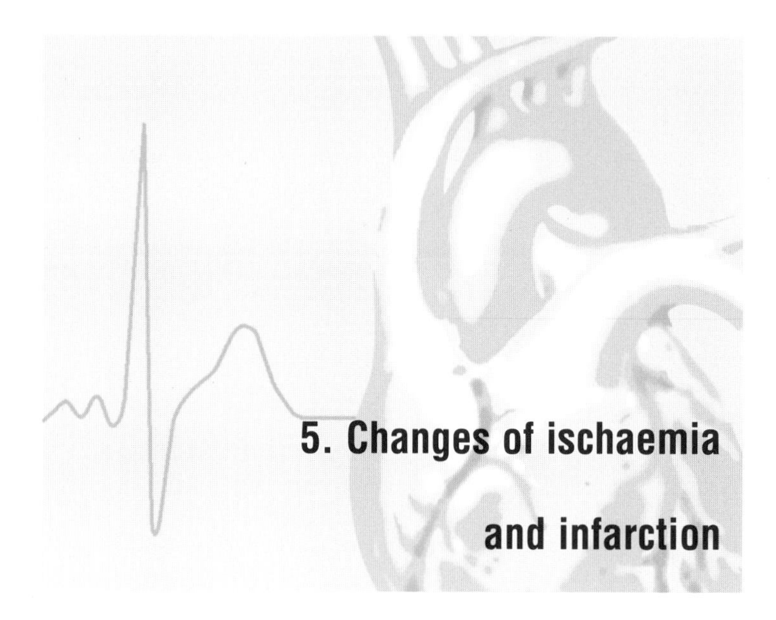

5. Changes of ischaemia and infarction

More ECGs are recorded, both in hospital practice and in the community, to assess coronary disease than for any other purpose. There is a problem with the use of electrocardiography in this role and it is important to realise this at the outset. The ECG records electrical activity from the myocardium, and abnormalities of this electrical activity will usually be present if the myocardium has been damaged by infarction or if acute ischaemia is present at the time of the recording. In many patients with coronary disease no myocardial abnormality is present, and normal electrical activity will be recorded. In these patients the problem lies not in the myocardium, but in the arteries that supply it with oxygenated blood. The resting ECG does not provide any direct evidence about the atheroma in the coronary arteries that may lead to myocardial ischaemia or infarction, even though such narrowings may be life-threatening.

The diagnosis of ischaemic heart disease has to be deduced indirectly by the effects that ischaemia produces on the electrical activation of the myocardium. It should be obvious, therefore, that a normal record does not exclude the presence of coronary artery disease - severe life-threatening coronary atheroma may be present yet the ECG may be entirely normal if no ischaemic damage to the myocardium has occurred.

Myocardial ischaemia and infarction are two manifestations of the same process; reduced myocardial oxygen supply caused, in most cases, by atheromatous narrowing or occlusion of the coronary arteries that supply the myocardium with oxygenated blood. The ECG changes of myocardial ischaemia that reflect hypoxia are most often seen during repolarisation; abnormalities of the ST segment and T wave result. The changes may be reversible if oxygenation is restored. If ischaemia becomes established the changes become more pronounced, and if infarction occurs permanent changes usually result. While changes in the ST segment and T wave also occur in myocardial infarction (and often provide the earliest ECG evidence that infarction is occurring), it is only the changes in the QRS complex that provide diagnostic evidence that infarction has actually taken place.

Infarction is the term used when muscle necrosis has occurred. Depolarisation of the ventricular myocardium is responsible for the QRS complex and it follows that infarction, with the loss of functioning myocardium, will modify these complexes. Ventricular depolarisation normally spreads from the endocardial surface to epicardium and will therefore be recorded as a positive R wave in an electrode recording from the epicardium or body surface. The loss of myocardium with infarction results in the loss of these positive electrical forces, and the consequent loss of R wave. Usually only the precordial leads can be used to diagnose the loss of R wave, as the R wave voltages in the limb leads are subject to other influences.

Infarcted myocardium is electrically 'dead' and therefore acts as a 'window' so that an electrode overlying the infarcted area will record depolarisation from the opposite wall of the heart. This depolarisation will also be travelling from endocardial to epicardial surface, and will be directed away from such an electrode; the result is a negative deflection on the ECG known as a pathological Q wave.

Changes in the ST segment and T wave occur during the early stages of infarction, and their appearance may fluctuate considerably. Elevation of the ST segment in leads overlying the area involved is usually the first sign and may develop very rapidly. The T waves in the same leads usually become inverted in the early stages. The permanent changes in the QRS complex produced by infarction (loss of R waves and the development of pathological Q waves) appear later and provide diagnostic information many years after the event. The ST segment returns to the isoelectric line in the days following the infarction while in time the T waves may resume their normal upright appearance.

Finally it must be remembered that ischaemia or infarction may cause changes in intracardiac rhythm or conduction; almost any arrhythmia or conduction disturbance may result.

Some of the electrocardiographic changes produced by coronary disease are illustrated in the following cases.

Case 4: Acute inferior infarction

This ECG was recorded from a 60-year-old man one hour after the onset of acute retrosternal pain. He had been treated for hypertension for several years but continued to smoke.

Sinus rhythm rate 60 per minute is present. The most striking abnormality is the marked elevation of the ST segment seen in the leads that record from the inferior surface of the heart (leads II, III and aVF). This is usually the first electrocardiographic manifestation of acute infarction, and may appear very rapidly - within minutes of the onset of chest pain. It is the characteristic ECG criterion for the administration of thrombolytic therapy. As infarction progresses, the ST segment returns towards the isoelectric line and changes in the QRS complex evolve. The ST elevation usually persists for a limited time, a few days at most, and the presence of this ST segment elevation with Q waves or reduced R waves usually means the infarct is relatively recent.

The ST segments in the lateral leads I and aVL show ST depression. These leads record from the opposite wall of the ventricle to that affected by the infarction, and the changes mirror those seen in the leads that record from the infarcted area.

Comment: This patient had risk factors for the development of atheromatous coronary disease, and sustained an inferior infarct.

ECG 4

Acute inferior infarction

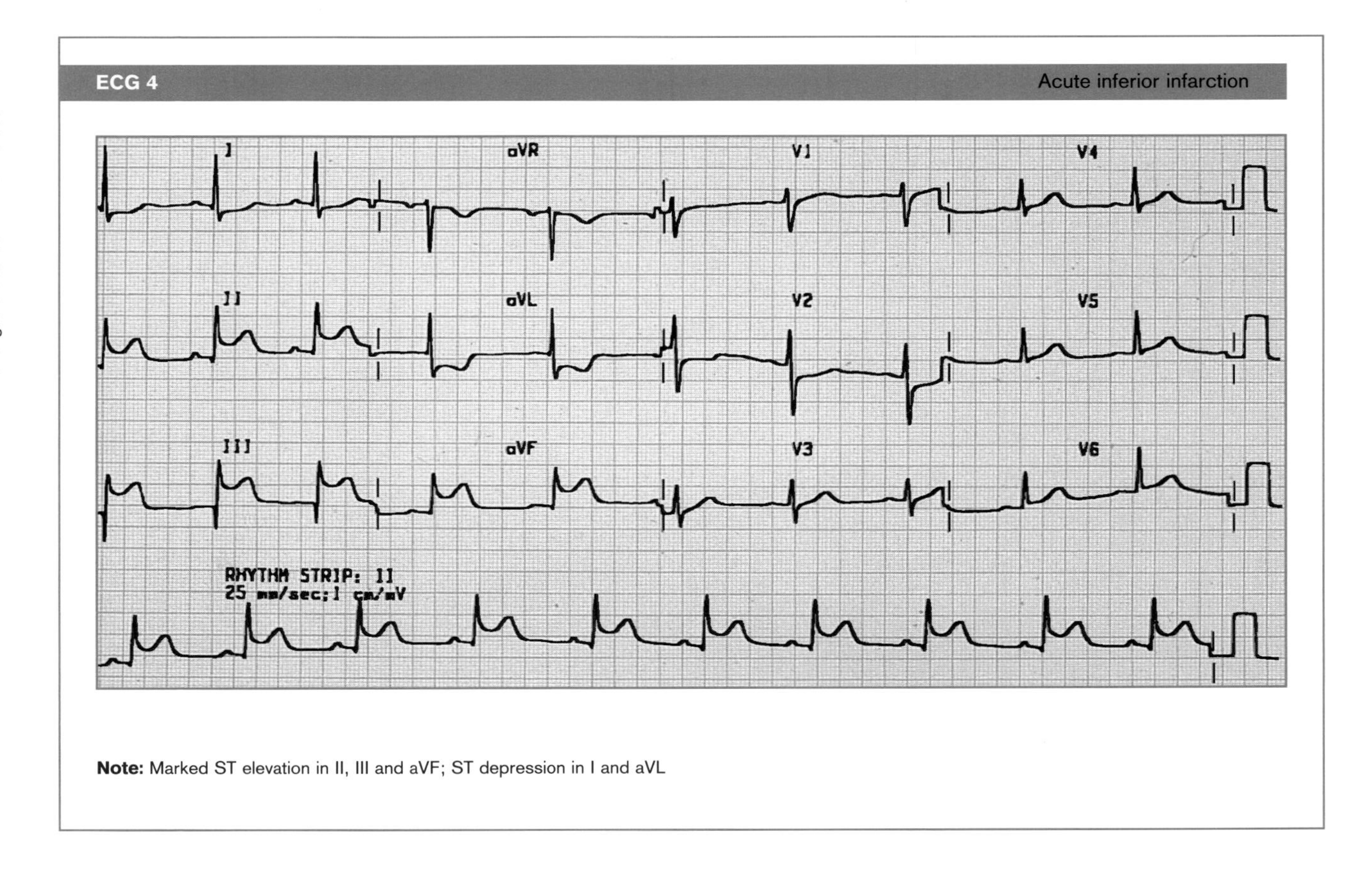

Note: Marked ST elevation in II, III and aVF; ST depression in I and aVL

Case 5: Acute inferior infarction, old anteroseptal infarction

This ECG was recorded in a 72-year-old man with diabetes who had developed acute chest pain. He had a history of anteroseptal infarction five years previously.

As in the previous example there is marked elevation of the ST segments in the leads recording from the inferior surface of the heart - II, III and aVF. Similarly, there is ST depression (and T wave inversion) in leads that record from the ventricular myocardium opposite the site of infarction - the anterior and lateral surface of the left ventricle (leads I, aVL, and V2 to V5). The pattern of R wave progression in the precordial leads is different from that seen in the normal ECGs (Cases 1 to 3). There is no smooth progression in the height of the R waves recorded by the precordial leads, and no significant R wave is recorded until V4. Larger R waves would have been expected in leads V2 and V3.

Comment: This patient had sustained an acute inferior myocardial infarct; the loss of R waves in the anteroseptal leads have remained as permanent evidence of previous infarction in this area.

ECG 5

Acute inferior infarction, old anteroseptal infarction

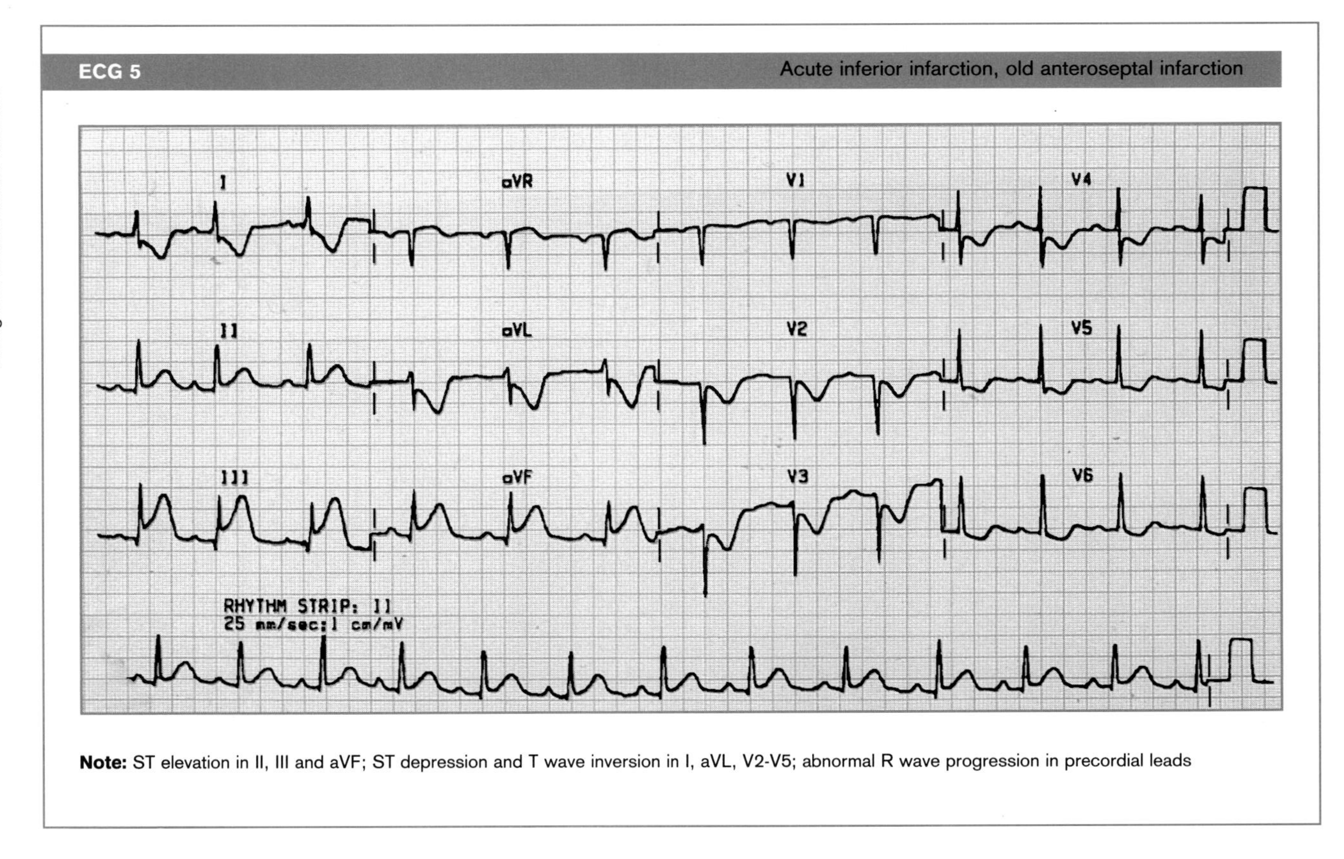

Note: ST elevation in II, III and aVF; ST depression and T wave inversion in I, aVL, V2-V5; abnormal R wave progression in precordial leads

Case 6: Acute anterior infarction, old inferior infarction

This ECG was recorded in a 54-year-old taxi driver who developed severe central chest pain. He had sustained an inferior infarction eight years previously when hyperlipidaemia was discovered. This had been treated but unfortunately he had continued to smoke. He was hypotensive, poorly perfused, and dyspnoeic.

There is marked ST elevation in the precordial leads V1 to V6 indicative of acute ischaemia in the anterior and lateral wall of the left ventricle. There are no significant R waves in any of the precordial leads, indicating that significant loss of myocardium has already occurred. There are pathological Q waves in leads III and aVF, which serve as evidence of the previous inferior infarction.

Comment: This patient had sustained an acute anterolateral infarct that caused damage to the left ventricle additional to that sustained at the time of the previous inferior infarction. The clinical appearance of cardiogenic shock reflected the impairment of ventricular function that resulted.

ECG 6

Acute anterior infarction, old inferior infarction

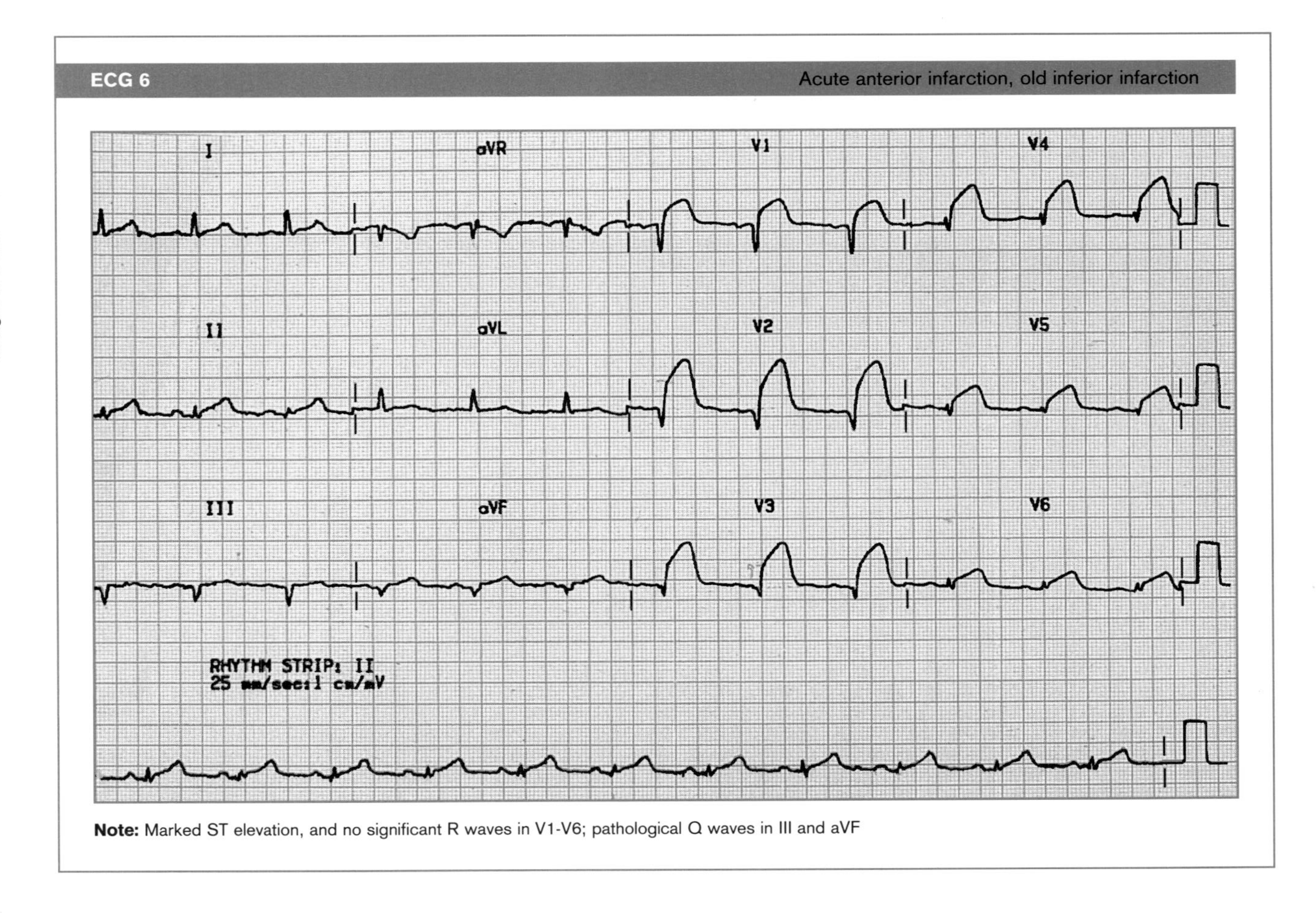

Note: Marked ST elevation, and no significant R waves in V1-V6; pathological Q waves in III and aVF

Case 7: Anterolateral infarction

This ECG was recorded from a 55-year-old man with a six-month history of angina that had been helped by treatment with nitrates and a beta-blocker. He developed similar, but more severe, pain while mowing the lawn. This did not pass with rest and the use of short-acting nitrates.

There is ST elevation in the precordial leads V2 to V6 signifying extensive anterolateral ischaemia. ST elevation is also present in the limb leads that record from the lateral surface of the heart: I and aVL. There is 'reciprocal' ST depression in leads aVR, III and aVF that record from the opposite wall of the heart. There are pathological Q waves in leads I, aVL, and V2 to V4, and there is marked loss of R wave in the precordial leads demonstrating that extensive infarction has occurred.

ECG 7

Anterolateral infarction

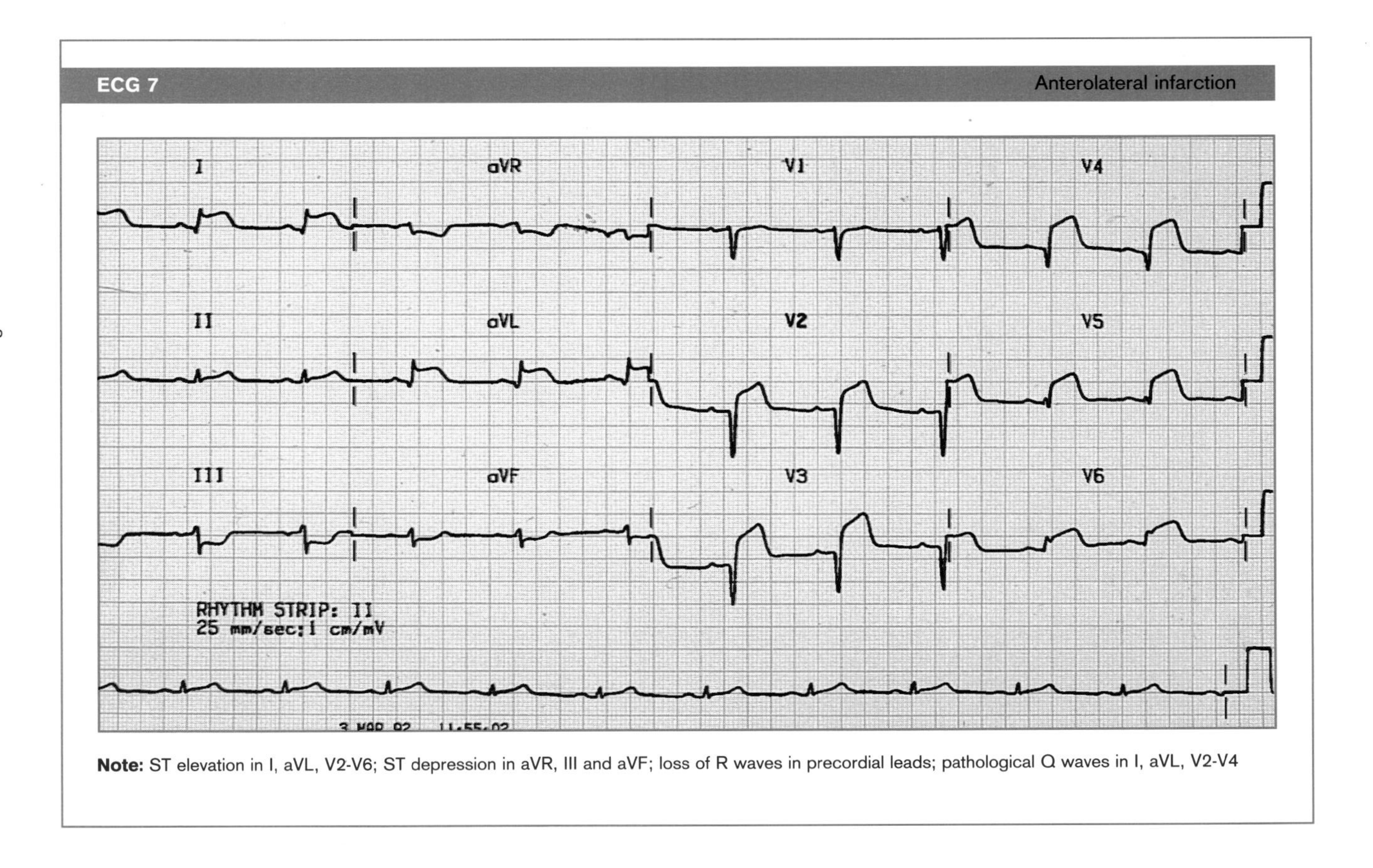

Note: ST elevation in I, aVL, V2-V6; ST depression in aVR, III and aVF; loss of R waves in precordial leads; pathological Q waves in I, aVL, V2-V4

Case 8: Recent anterior infarction

This ECG was recorded from a patient with an acute anterior infarct five days after admission to the coronary care unit.

There are prominent Q waves in the precordial leads V1 to V5, and loss of R wave has also occurred in the precordial leads - no R wave is recorded until V5. These are diagnostic features of myocardial infarction. At the time the ECG was recorded the ST segments were returning towards the isoelectric line but ST elevation was still present in leads V2 to V5. The T waves are inverted in the limb leads (I and aVL) and the precordial leads (V2 to V5) that record from the anterolateral surface of the heart.

Comment: The ECG shows several of the changes that evolve during myocardial infarction. Q waves and loss of R wave provide definite evidence that infarction has taken place. T wave inversion occurs in the leads that record from the area of infarction, i.e. the same leads as show ST elevation in the initial phase. T wave inversion is, however, a later sign and usually occurs after ST elevation is well established. As the ST segments return to the baseline the T waves typically show a pattern of symmetrical inversion. T wave inversion may be permanent, but as recovery takes place (usually after some months) the T waves may revert to their upright position.

ECG 8

Recent anterior infarction

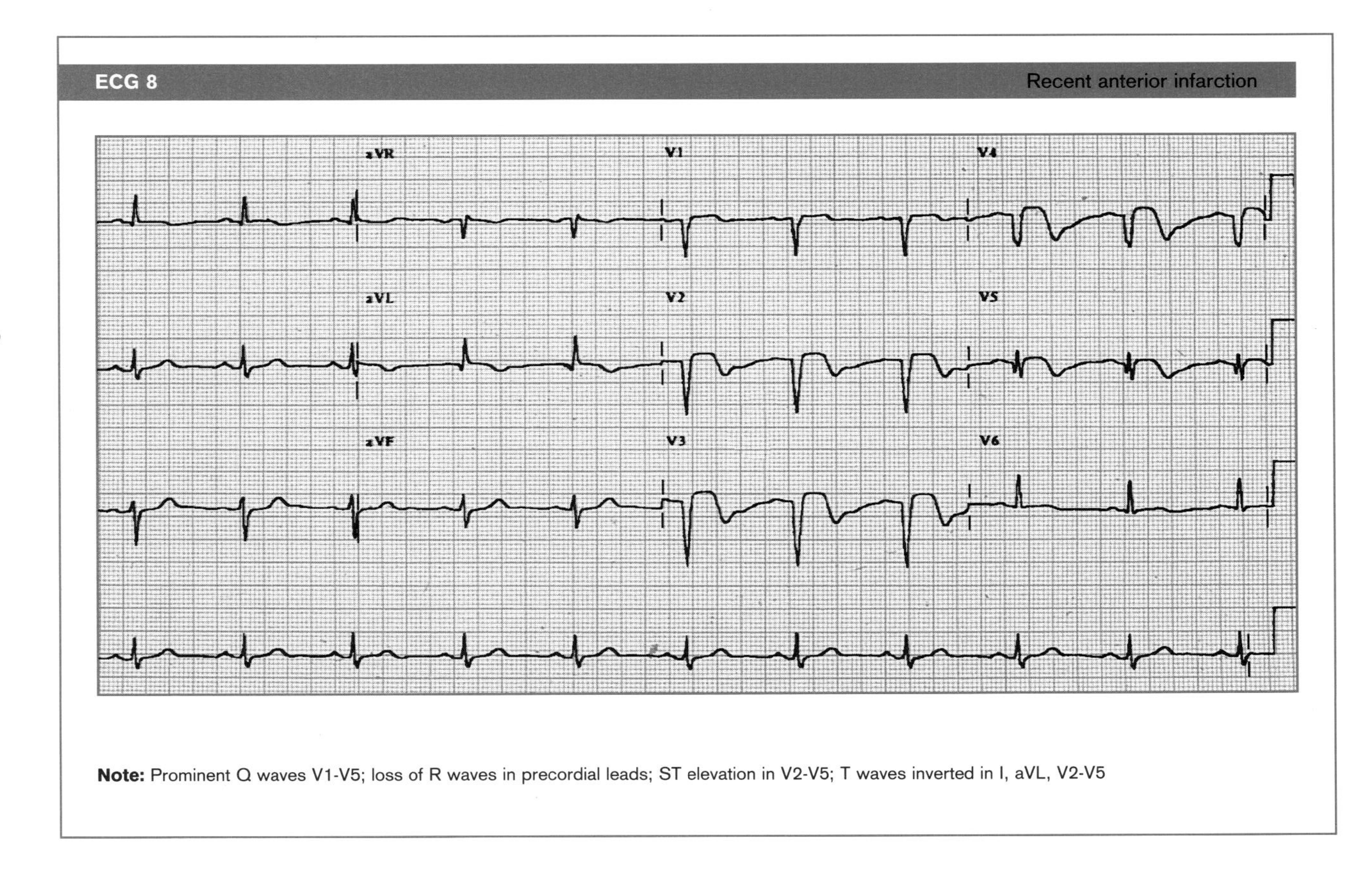

Note: Prominent Q waves V1-V5; loss of R waves in precordial leads; ST elevation in V2-V5; T waves inverted in I, aVL, V2-V5

Case 9: Recent anterolateral infarction

This ECG was recorded from a 67-year-old woman one week after admission to the coronary care unit with an anterior infarction.

Loss of R waves has occurred in the precordial leads and pathological Q waves are present in leads V4 to V6 demonstrating that infarction has taken place. Note that R waves are present in V1 to V3 so that the complexes are rS waves, not QS waves as in V4. The ST segments are still elevated in leads V1 to V5, and deep symmetrical T inversion has occurred in leads V2 to V5. The T waves are also inverted in leads I and aVL , and in leads II, III and aVF.

Comment: As the ST segment elevation of acute infarction resolves, the T waves in the area affected by infarction often become inverted, and may show a pattern of deep symmetrical inversion; this is well illustrated in V4 and V5. The appearance is typical of recent anterior infarction.

ECG 9

Recent anterolateral infarction

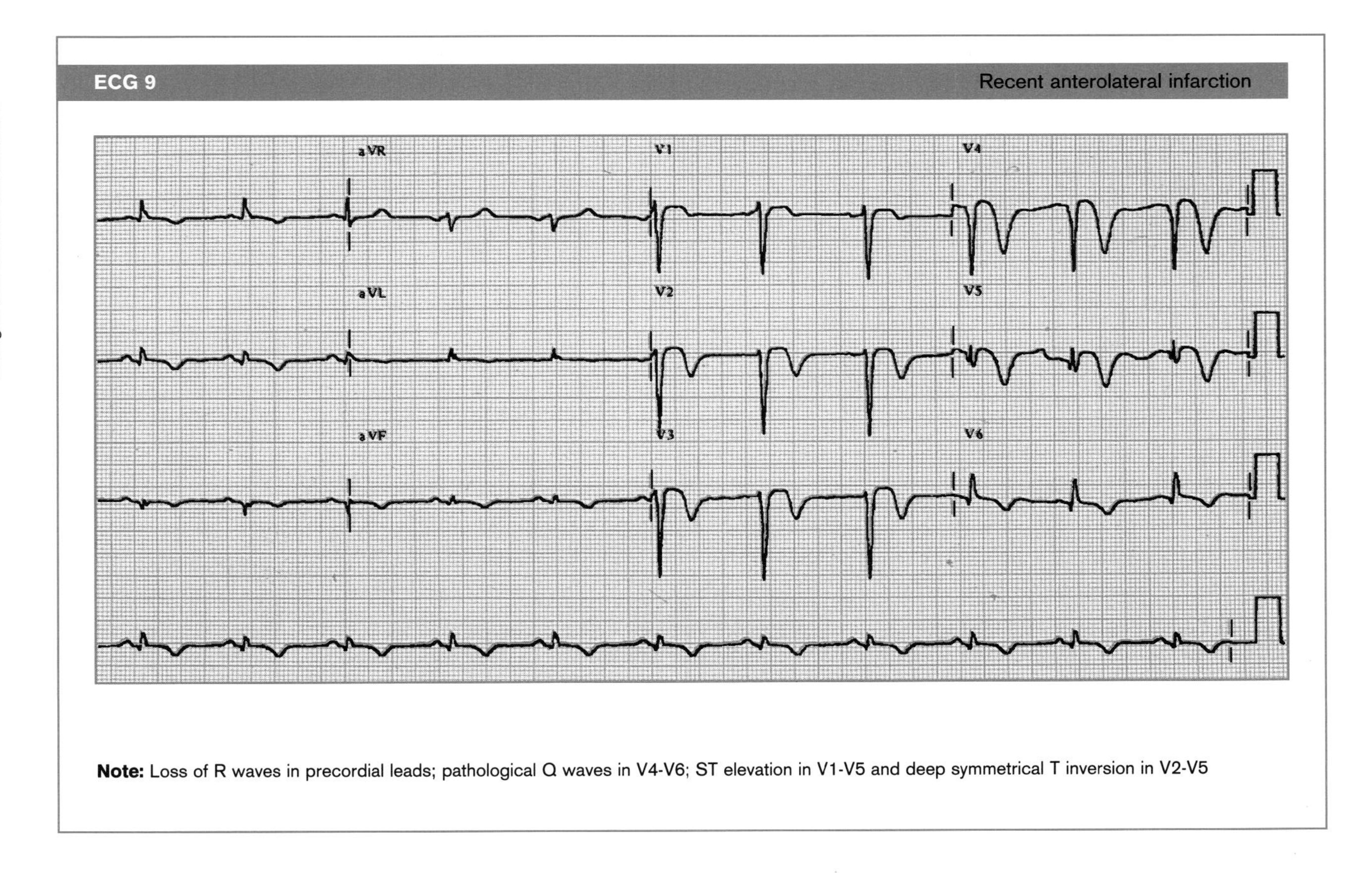

Note: Loss of R waves in precordial leads; pathological Q waves in V4-V6; ST elevation in V1-V5 and deep symmetrical T inversion in V2-V5

Case 10: Acute inferolateral infarction

This ECG was recorded from a 46-year-old man admitted to the coronary care unit following the onset of retrosternal chest pain.

ST elevation is present in leads I, II, aVF and aVL, and leads V3 to V6, indicating acute ischaemia. A pathological Q wave is present in aVL, being 40 msec in duration and more than 25% of the height of the R wave that follows. The Q waves in V5 and V6 are less than 40 msec in duration but are more than 25% of the height of the following R wave, and also indicate that infarction has occurred.

Comment: ST segment elevation is present in leads that record from the inferior and lateral surface of the heart. The presence of Q waves in the lateral leads indicates that infarction has taken place in this area. The R waves in the precordial leads are well preserved, and this record does not, therefore, show any loss of myocardium from the anterior surface of the heart.

ECG 10 Acute inferolateral infarction

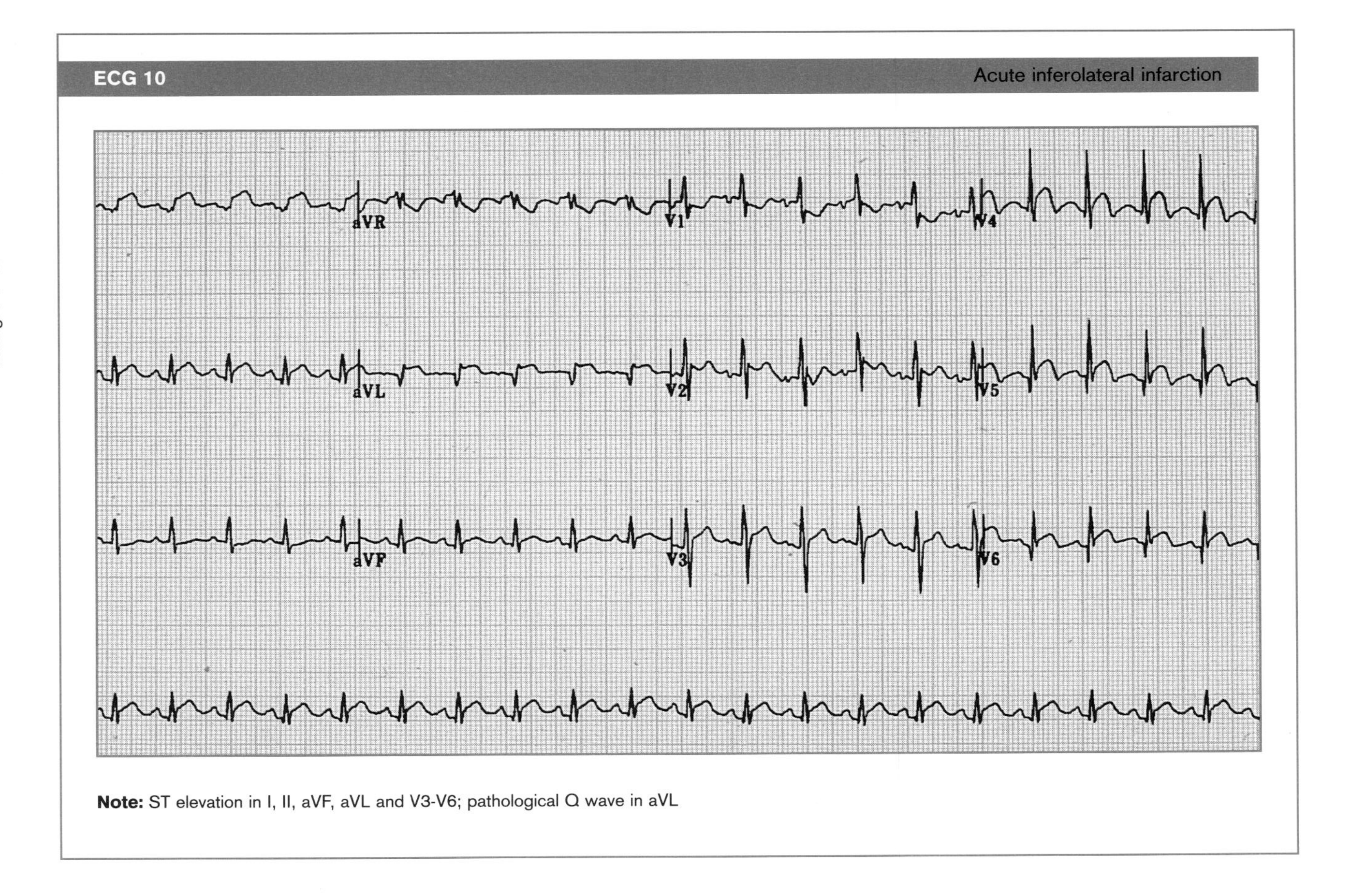

Note: ST elevation in I, II, aVF, aVL and V3-V6; pathological Q wave in aVL

Case 11: Inferior infarction with true posterior infarction

This ECG was recorded in a 19-year-old man admitted to hospital for unrelated reasons. He had complained of chest pain four days before admission and the ECG was recorded because of this.

There are pathological Q waves in the inferior leads - II, III and aVF. The prominent Q waves in V5 and V6 are more difficult to define; in V5 the Q wave is less than 25% of the height of the following R wave and less than 40 msec in duration, and is therefore best considered non-pathological. The Q wave in V6, however, is more than 25% of the height of the following R wave and is at least 40 msec in duration; it has the same significance as the Q waves in the inferior leads. The T waves are inverted in the same leads as those with pathological Q waves, providing further evidence of infarction in the inferolateral region.

In leads V1 and V2 there are tall R waves exceeding 40 msec in duration, and in addition there are tall peaked T waves in leads V1, V2 and V3. These are the typical changes of true posterior wall infarction.

Comment: Inferior wall infarction used to be termed posterior wall infarction (despite the fact that this is not anatomically correct). For this reason infarction of the anatomical posterior wall is often termed true posterior infarction. True posterior infarction is unusual and is often associated with inferior infarction as both areas are frequently supplied by the same coronary artery.

No lead in the standard 12-lead ECG records from the true posterior surface of the heart. Leads V1 and V2 record reciprocal changes from the opposite wall of the heart. The tall R waves are the equivalent of the Q wave recorded from leads overlying the infarcted area, and the tall peaked T wave is the reciprocal of the deep symmetrical T wave inversion. ST segment changes in V1 and V2 may also be seen.

In this case the cardiac enzymes were elevated in a pattern typical of acute infarction. Subsequent coronary angiography demonstrated normal coronary vessels, but hypokinesia was observed in the inferior and posterior wall of the left ventricle. Not all myocardial infarcts are due to atheromatous coronary disease - emboli may occur, and occasionally arteritis or spasm of the vessels may be responsible. The precise cause in this patient remained unproved.

ECG 11

Inferior infarction with true posterior infarction

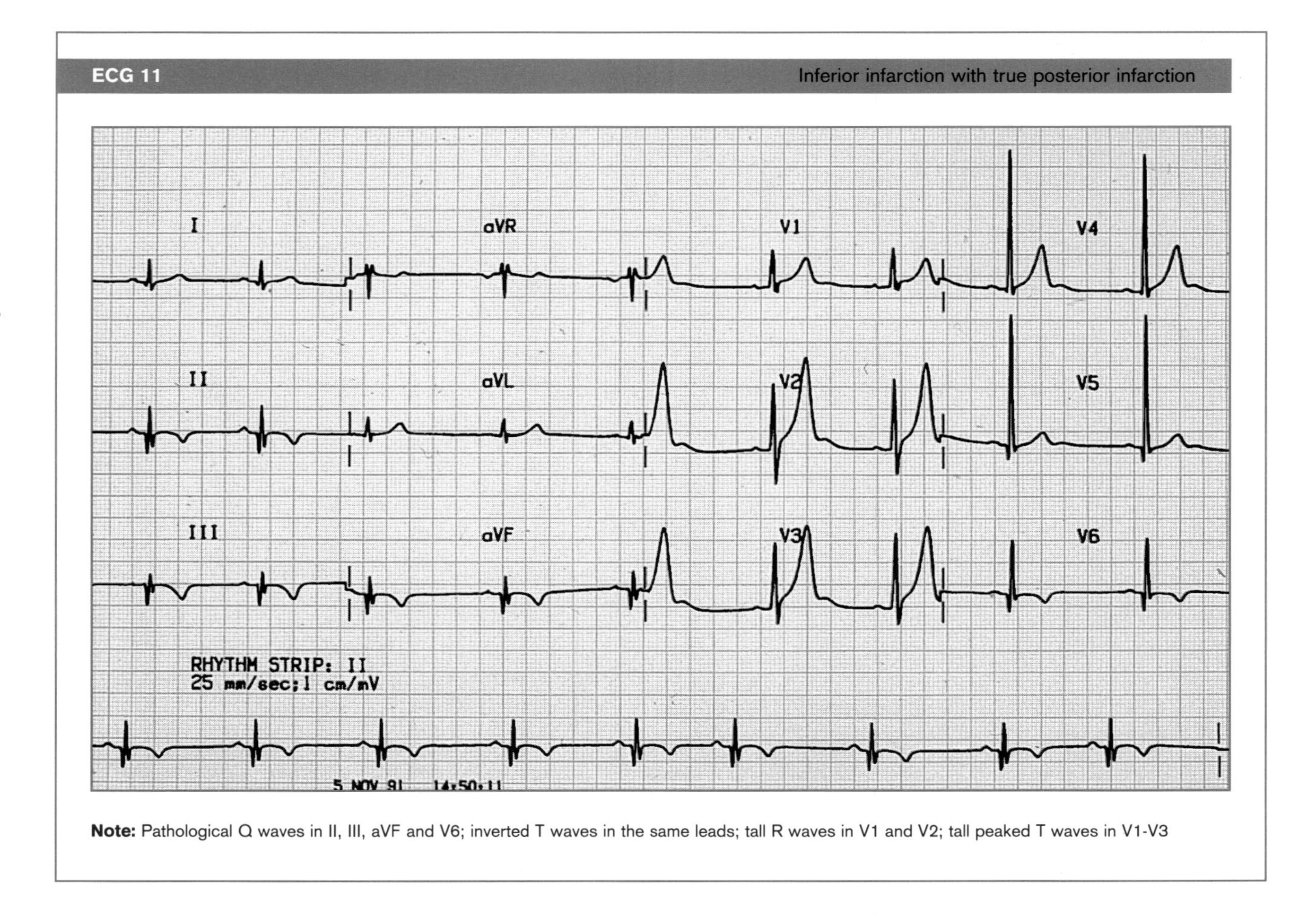

Note: Pathological Q waves in II, III, aVF and V6; inverted T waves in the same leads; tall R waves in V1 and V2; tall peaked T waves in V1-V3

Case 12: Old inferior myocardial infarction

This ECG was recorded in a 78-year-old man about to undergo prostatic surgery. He had no cardiac symptoms and had no recollection of any significant episode of chest pain.

The ECG is abnormal. There are pathological Q waves in leads II, III and aVF, and the T waves are inverted in these leads. These signs are typical of inferior myocardial infarction having occurred at some time, but it is not possible from the ECG to say when this happened. Myocardial ischaemia may also be responsible for the flattened T waves in leads V5 and V6, but there are no Q waves to indicate infarction in these leads.

Comment: Myocardial infarction may be painless, and this type of infarction is often described as a silent infarct. Painless infarction occurs particularly in elderly people.

ECG 12 Old inferior myocardial infarction

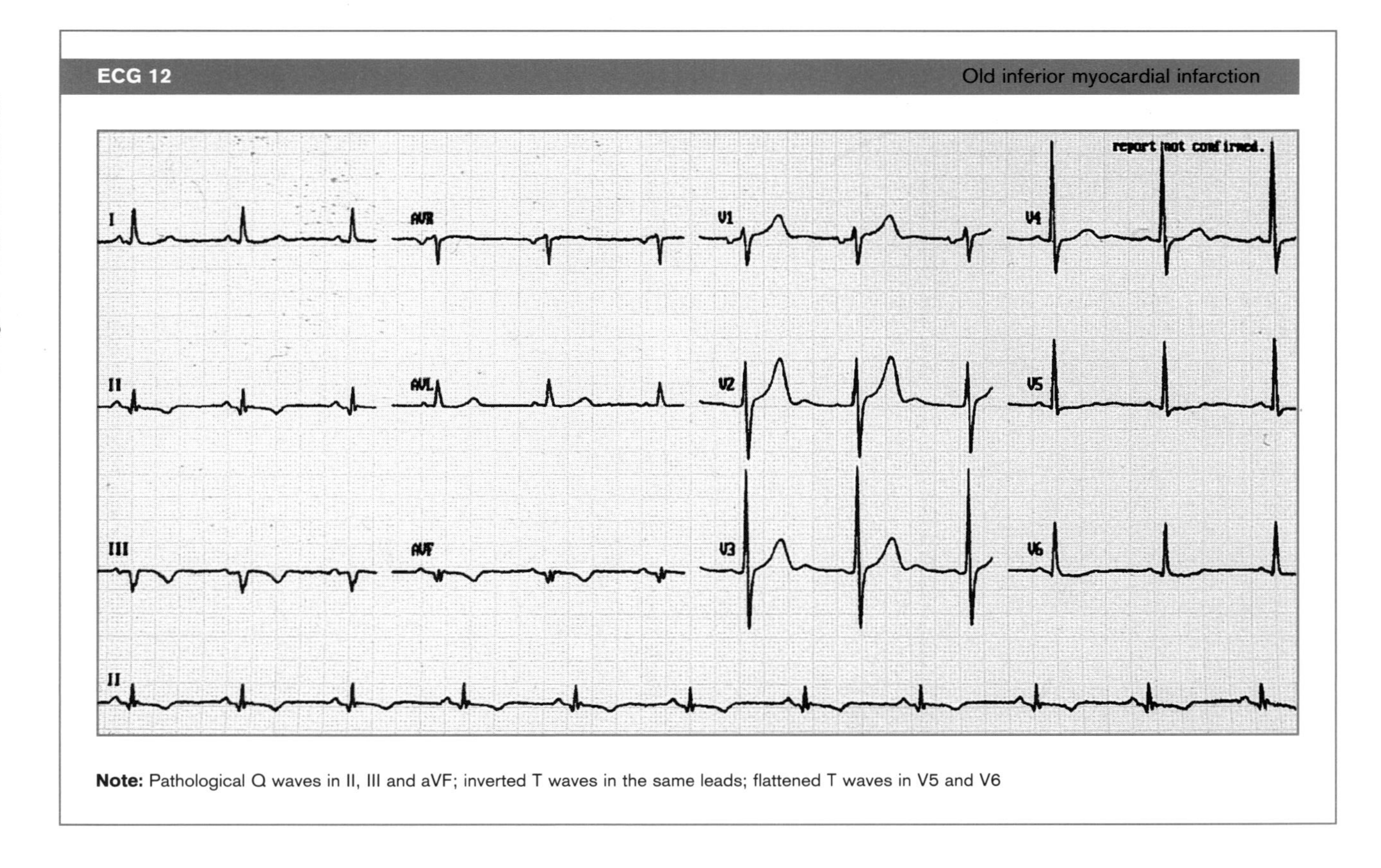

Note: Pathological Q waves in II, III and aVF; inverted T waves in the same leads; flattened T waves in V5 and V6

Case 13: Old anterolateral infarction

This ECG was recorded in a 54-year-old man two years after he had been admitted to hospital with an anterior infarction. In the weeks before this recording was made he had begun to experience angina on fairly modest exertion.

There are pathological Q waves in the precordial leads recording from the anterolateral surface of the heart - leads V2, V3, V4, V5 and V6. There has been loss of R waves in the precordial leads V2 to V5; no R wave at all is recorded until V5 where a small one is seen. The R wave in V6 is reasonable, demonstrating the presence of viable myocardium in this area. The T waves are inverted in leads V5 and V6, and are also flattened or inverted in the inferior leads II, III and aVF. There are also pathological Q waves in leads I and aVL, which record from the lateral surface of the heart. The ST segments in leads V2 to V4 remain elevated (more than 1 mm above the isoelectric line).

Comment: The appearances are of old anterolateral infarction. Two years after the event the T waves in V2 to V4 have regained their normal upright appearance. The T waves are inverted in leads recording from the inferolateral surface of the heart - II, III, aVF, V5 and V6. These appearances may represent continuing ischaemia in this area. The ST segments have remained elevated in the precordial leads at a stage when they would usually have returned to normal. This appearance of persistent ST elevation is sometimes indicative of a left ventricular aneurysm. This was confirmed by cardiac catheterisation, and coronary angiography showed occlusion of the left anterior descending coronary artery with significant stenoses in the right and circumflex vessels.

ECG 13 — Old anterolateral infarction

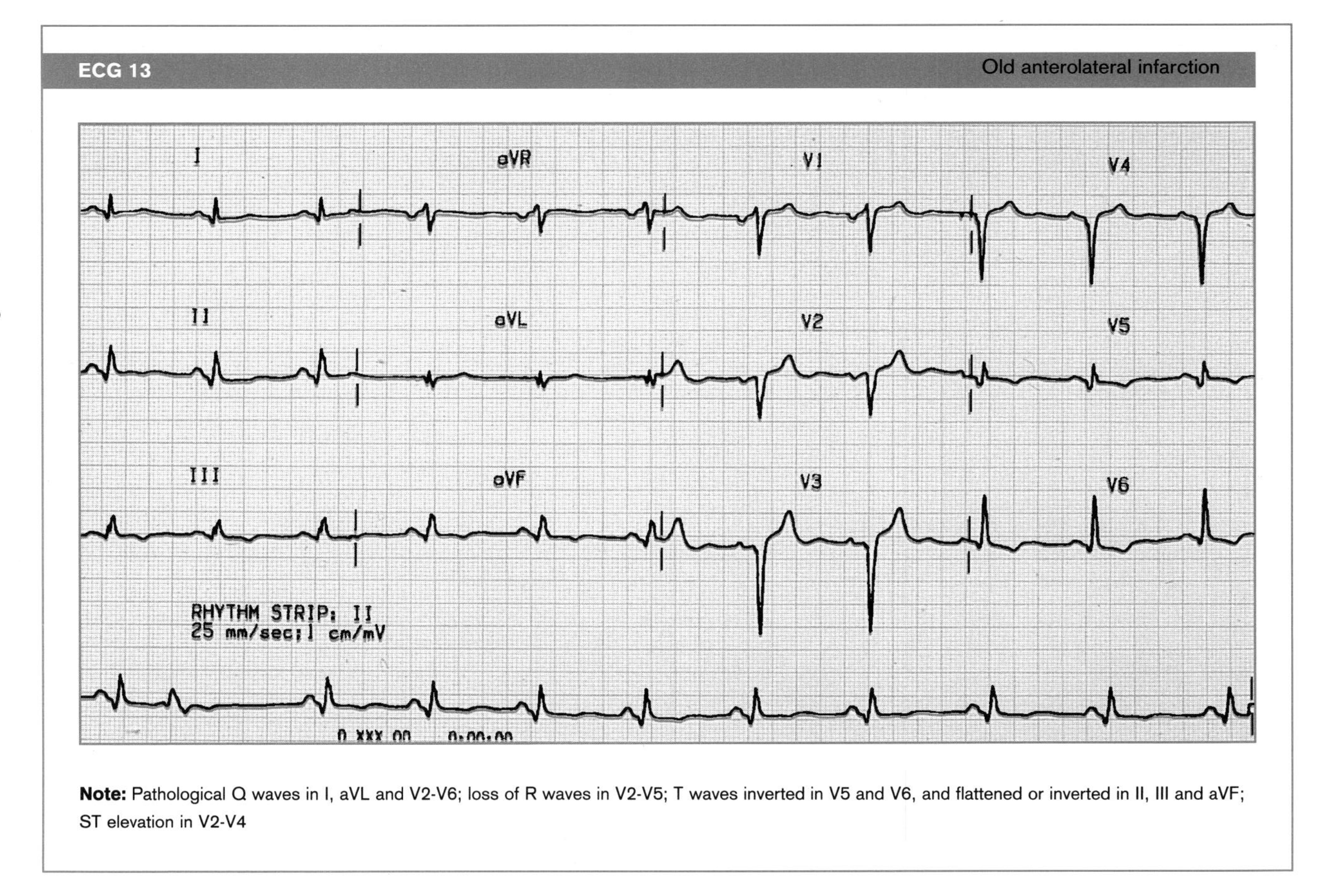

Note: Pathological Q waves in I, aVL and V2-V6; loss of R waves in V2-V5; T waves inverted in V5 and V6, and flattened or inverted in II, III and aVF; ST elevation in V2-V4

Case 14: Subendocardial infarction

This ECG was recorded in a 54-year-old woman admitted to the coronary care unit with the clinical picture of acute myocardial infarction.

Sinus bradycardia (rate 42 per minute) is present. The ECG shows widespread ST depression and T wave inversion. The changes are most marked in the anterolateral precordial leads V2 to V5. The T waves are also abnormal in all the limb leads, being biphasic or inverted. There are no pathological Q waves - the small q waves seen in leads I and aVL are less than 40 msec duration.

Comment: The ECG is compatible with acute ischaemia, but the appearances could also be caused by subendocardial infarction. It is impossible to distinguish between the two from the ECG alone. Changes produced by ischaemia alone tend to be short-lived, and the diagnosis of subendocardial infarction is made by recording serial records showing persisting changes. The cardiac enzymes were also raised in this case, providing confirmation of the diagnosis. Subendocardial infarction involves a partial thickness of the myocardium, and sufficient viable myocardium remains to generate anteriorly directed electrical forces. These prevent the exploring electrode from recording a purely negative Q wave from the ventricular wall opposite the area of infarction.

ECG 14 Subendocardial infarction

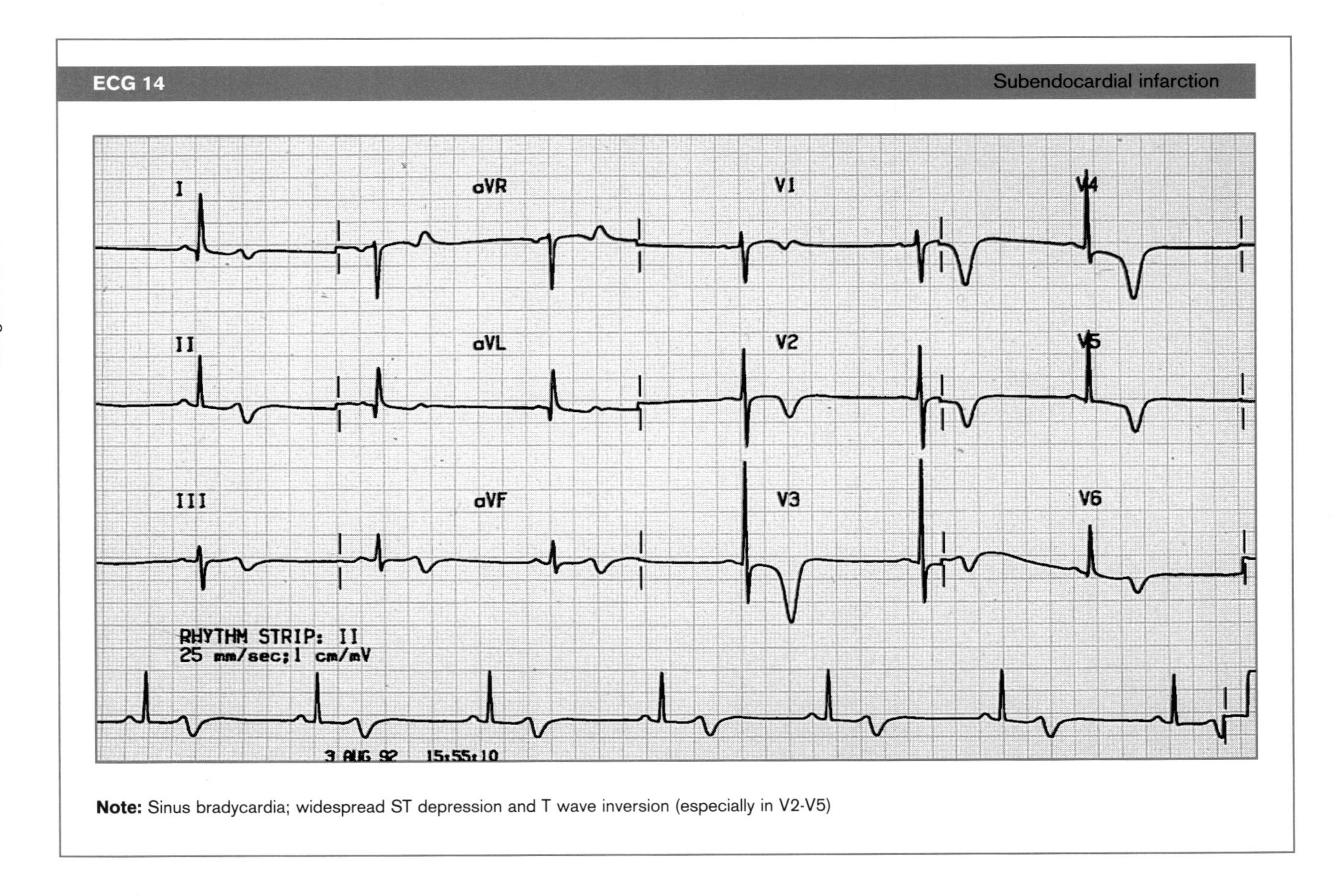

Note: Sinus bradycardia; widespread ST depression and T wave inversion (especially in V2-V5)

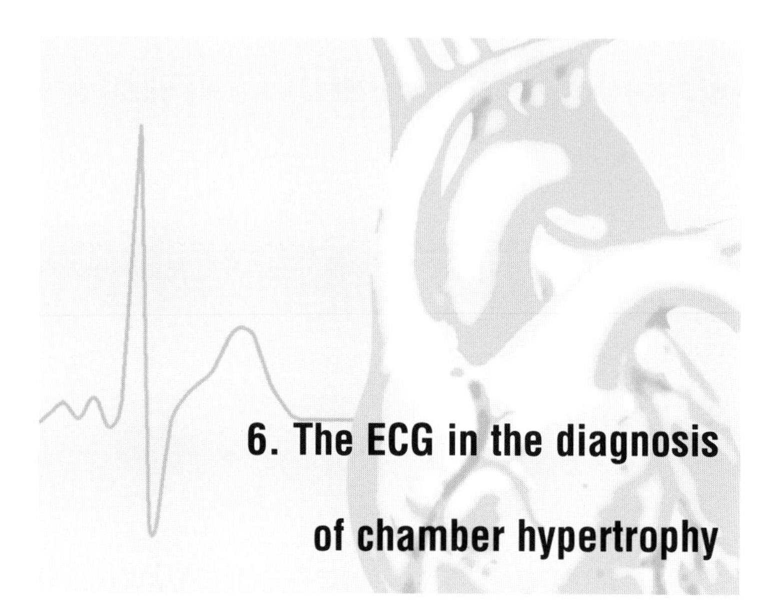

6. The ECG in the diagnosis of chamber hypertrophy

Each cardiac chamber contributes to the deflections recorded on the ECG during the cardiac cycle. Cardiac chamber hypertrophy may be detectable on the ECG either because the larger muscle mass generates a greater voltage than normal, or because delayed spread of depolarisation through the increased muscle mass results in prolongation of the complex for which it is responsible.

Ventricular hypertrophy

In ventricular hypertrophy the typical pattern recorded shows:

1. Increased voltages - a tall R wave in leads recording from the epicardial surface of the hypertrophied ventricle. Deep S or

QS waves are recorded from cavity leads or leads overlying the non-hypertrophied ventricle.

2. Prolongation of the QRS interval - but not beyond 100 msec, when bundle branch block would be diagnosed. Bundle branch block is not a feature of ventricular hypertrophy *per se* but may coexist with hypertrophy and complicate interpretation.

3. Prolongation of the ventricular activation time (VAT). This is a measure of the time taken for the impulse to travel from endocardium to epicardium. The measurement is taken from the start of the Q wave to the peak of the R wave, and is best made in V5 or V6 in left ventricular hypertrophy (LVH) when prolongation to 50 msec may be seen. In right ventricular hypertrophy (RVH) the measurement should be made in a right ventricular lead that shows a tall R wave, often V1. In RVH the VAT typically exceeds 30 msec.

4. Abnormalities in repolarisation. ST segment depression and T wave inversion are often seen in leads recording from the epicardial surface of the hypertrophied ventricle. ST elevation and upright T waves are frequently seen in leads overlying the non-hypertrophied ventricle.

Left ventricular hypertrophy

No internationally recognised criteria exist for the diagnosis of ventricular hypertrophy, but the following are suggested to help the diagnosis of LVH:

1. The R wave in V5 or V6 exceeds 27 mm.
2. The S wave in V1 or V2 exceeds 25 mm.

3. The sum of the R wave in V5 or V6 and the S wave in V1 exceeds 35 mm. An alternative to this is that the sum of the tallest R wave and the deepest S wave exceeds 40 mm.
4. The R wave in aVL exceeds 13 mm.
5. The R wave in aVF exceeds 20 mm when the frontal plane QRS axis is vertical.
6. The ventricular activation time (VAT) is 50 msec or more.
7. ST segment depression and T wave inversion are present in leads facing the left ventricle in association with voltage criteria.

The more criteria fulfilled, the more accurate the ECG diagnosis, but it is important to remember that significant ventricular hypertrophy may be present without ECG evidence of its presence.

Right ventricular hypertrophy

The following criteria suggest RVH:

1. A dominant R wave is present in V1. The R:S ratio should be 1 or more, or the R wave should reach 7 mm.
2. Right axis deviation of +110 degrees or more.
3. The sum of the voltage of the R wave in V1 and the S wave in V6 is 10 mm or more.
4. An S wave deeper than the height of the R wave in V6, or persistent S waves in leads facing the left ventricle (I, aVL, V5 and V6).
5. ST/T wave changes in leads overlying the right ventricle (V1 to V3).

Other causes of right axis deviation or a dominant R wave in V1 (the Wolff-Parkinson-White syndrome, true posterior infarction and right bundle branch block) must be absent.

Atrial hypertrophy

Left atrial hypertrophy

Conduction delay through hypertrophied muscle results in prolongation of the P wave; this is usually best seen in lead II, and a P wave duration of 120 msec suggests left atrial hypertrophy (LAH). The increased voltage is usually best recorded in V1 where the terminal negative component of the biphasic P wave normally seen in this lead is increased in amplitude (to more than 1 mm). Sometimes an M-shaped appearance is seen in lead II, reflecting separation of the contributions made by each atrium to the P wave. The conduction delay and increased voltage accentuate the left atrial contribution which is the second peak of the M.

Right atrial hypertrophy

Right atrial depolarisation is normally complete before depolarisation of the left atrium, and even in the presence of right atrial hypertrophy (RAH) the total duration of the P wave is not increased. The increased voltage generated during depolarisation of the hypertrophied right atrium may be recorded as an increase in P wave amplitude, best seen in lead II (and often leads III and aVF), and as an increase in the initial positive deflection of the P wave in V1.

The P wave should not exceed 2.5 mm in height in lead II, and an increase above this suggests the presence of RAH. Tall peaked

P waves (often 3 mm or more) are characteristically seen in lead II and the other inferior leads. This appearance is often termed P pulmonale because of the frequent association of RAH with pulmonary hypertension.

The following examples illustrate many of the ECG features of cardiac chamber hypertrophy.

Case 15: Left ventricular hypertrophy on voltage criteria

This ECG was recorded from a 70-year-old woman with long-standing hypertension.

The voltage criteria described for LVH are easily met, and the VAT is prolonged to 50 msec.

Comment: When no ST segment or T wave changes are recorded, it is usually better to say that the voltage criteria for LVH are met rather than to diagnose hypertrophy. Tall R waves may be recorded under normal circumstances in young fit individuals with thin chest walls.

ECG 15 Left ventricular hypertrophy on voltage criteria

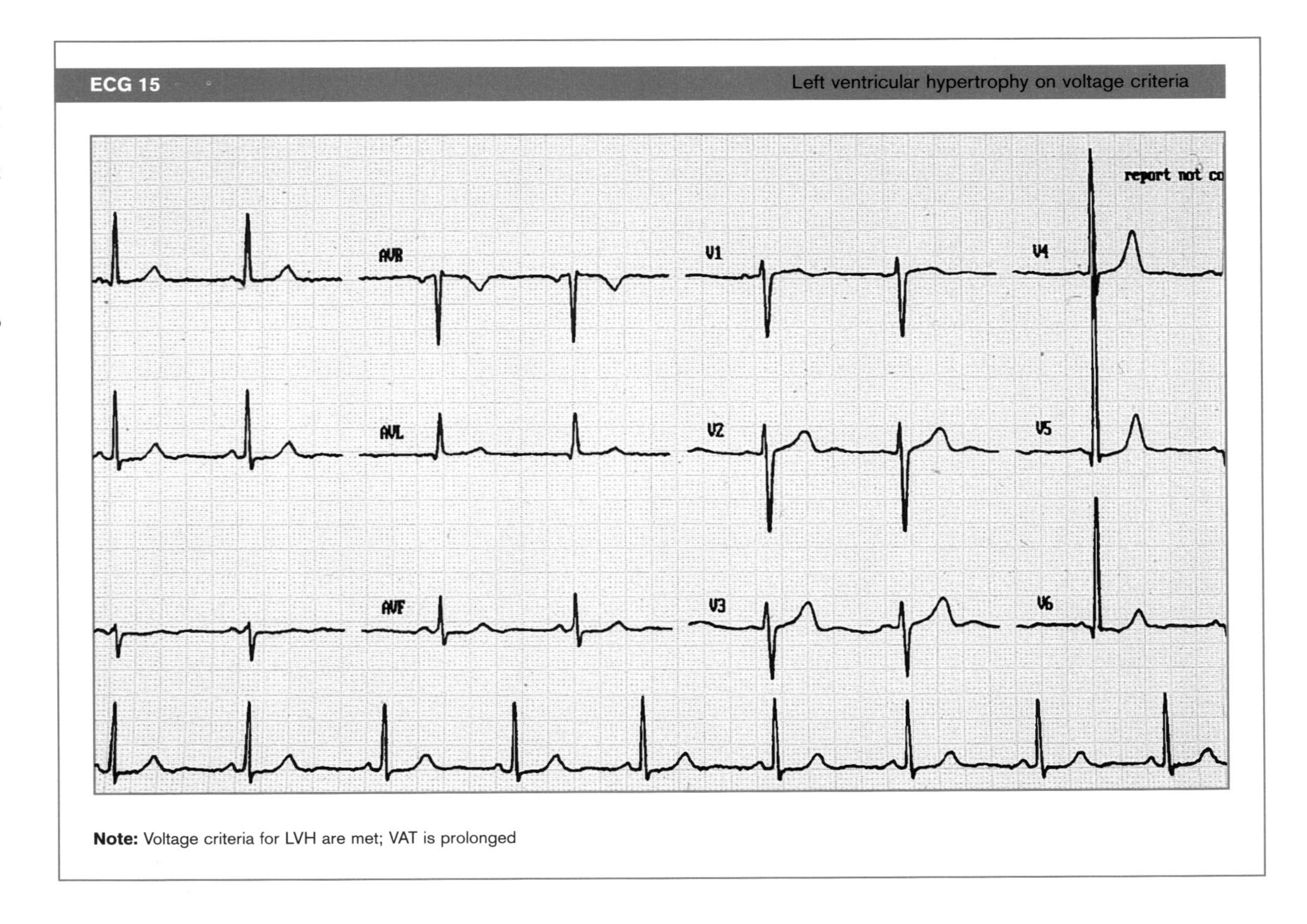

Note: Voltage criteria for LVH are met; VAT is prolonged

Case 16: Left ventricular hypertrophy with recent inferior infarction

This ECG was recorded in a 60-year-old man four days after admission with an uncomplicated inferior infarct. He had been hypertensive for many years.

The voltage criteria described for LVH are met. In addition there are pathological Q waves in the inferior leads (III and aVF), and ST segment elevation is present reflecting the recent infarction in this area. The terminal negative component of the P wave in V1 is 40 msec in duration suggesting left atrial hypertrophy.

The ST segments are depressed and the T waves are inverted in leads I, aVL, V5 and V6. It is not possible to say from the ECG alone whether these changes reflect left ventricular hypertrophy or ischaemia (or both).

ECG 16

Left ventricular hypertrophy with recent inferior infarction

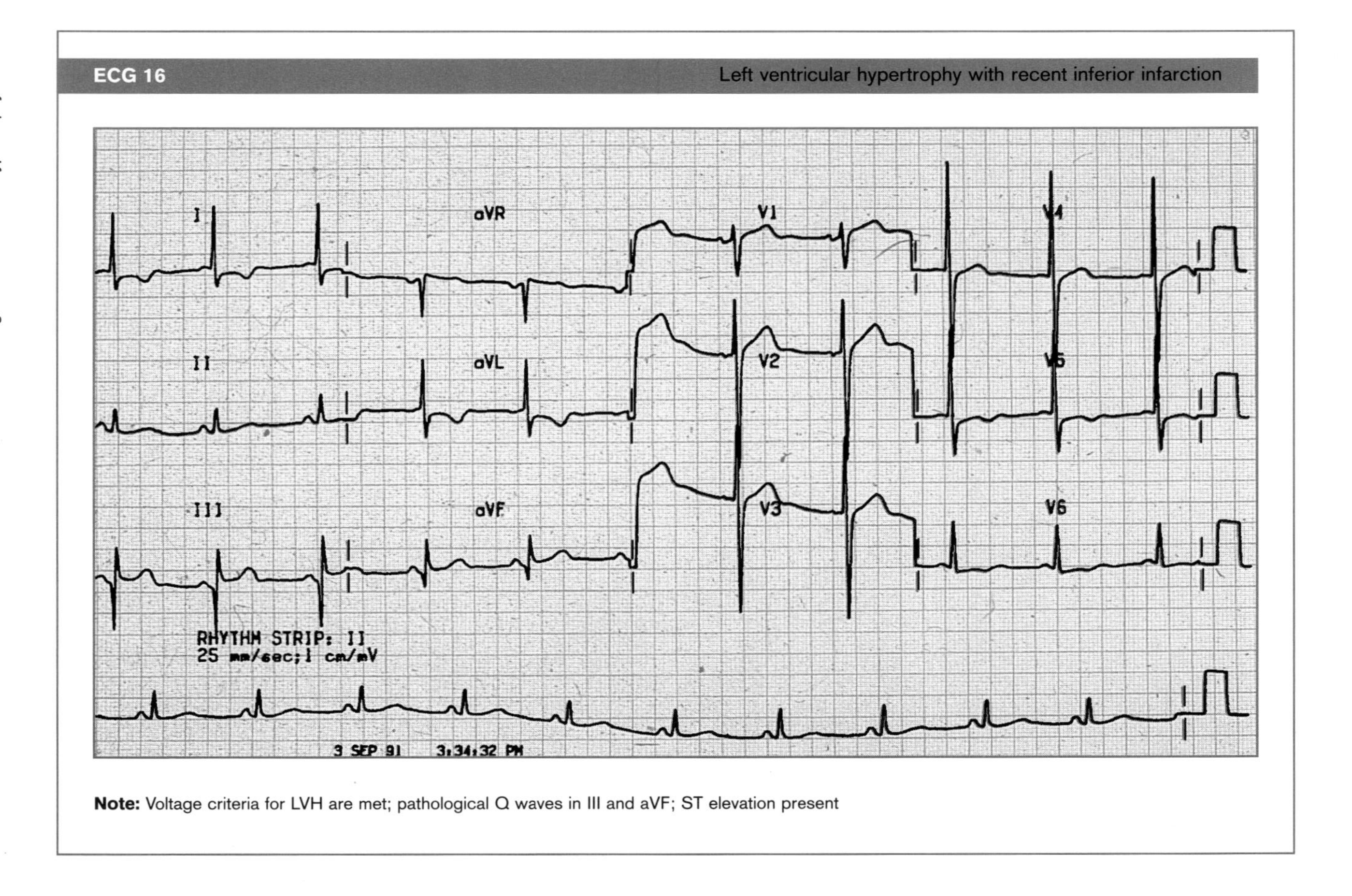

Note: Voltage criteria for LVH are met; pathological Q waves in III and aVF; ST elevation present

Case 17: Left ventricular hypertrophy with anterior infarction and inferior infarction

This ECG was recorded in a 74-year-old man with mild aortic valve disease; he had also been treated for hypertension for several years.

Pathological Q waves are present in the inferior leads II, III and aVF, indicating that infarction has occurred in this area. Pathological Q waves are also present in the anteroseptal leads V2, V3, and V4, indicating that infarction has also occurred in this area. The lack of R wave progression in the precordial leads also supports this diagnosis. The ST segments are depressed and the T waves are inverted in the lateral leads I, aVL, V5 and V6. The ST segments are elevated in the inferior leads.

The negative terminal part of the P wave in lead V1 is greater than 1 mm deep and 1 mm (40 msec) wide, and the P wave in lead II is prolonged to 120 msec and shows an M-shaped appearance. These features suggest left atrial hypertrophy.

The PR interval is 220 msec and is therefore prolonged above the upper limit of normal. First-degree AV block is present.

Comment: Significant LVH had been demonstrated on echocardiography and was thought to be due to a combination of hypertensive and valvular heart disease. The only voltage criteria for LVH met is that the R wave in aVL exceeds 13 mm. ECGs recorded before his anterior infarct easily satisfied the voltage criteria for LVH, but the loss of R wave in the precordial leads that occurred at the time of infarction made the subsequent diagnosis of LVH from the ECG less secure. Left atrial hypertrophy is present - this often accompanies left ventricular hypertrophy.

The ST segment changes are difficult to interpret; the inferior infarct was not recent, and the ST elevation in the inferior leads may be a reciprocal change to the depression seen in leads I and aVL. The changes might reflect hypertrophy, but as ischaemia may also affect the ST segment and T waves it is better not to be too specific about the origin of these changes.

ECG 17 Left ventricular hypertrophy with anterior infarction and inferior infarction

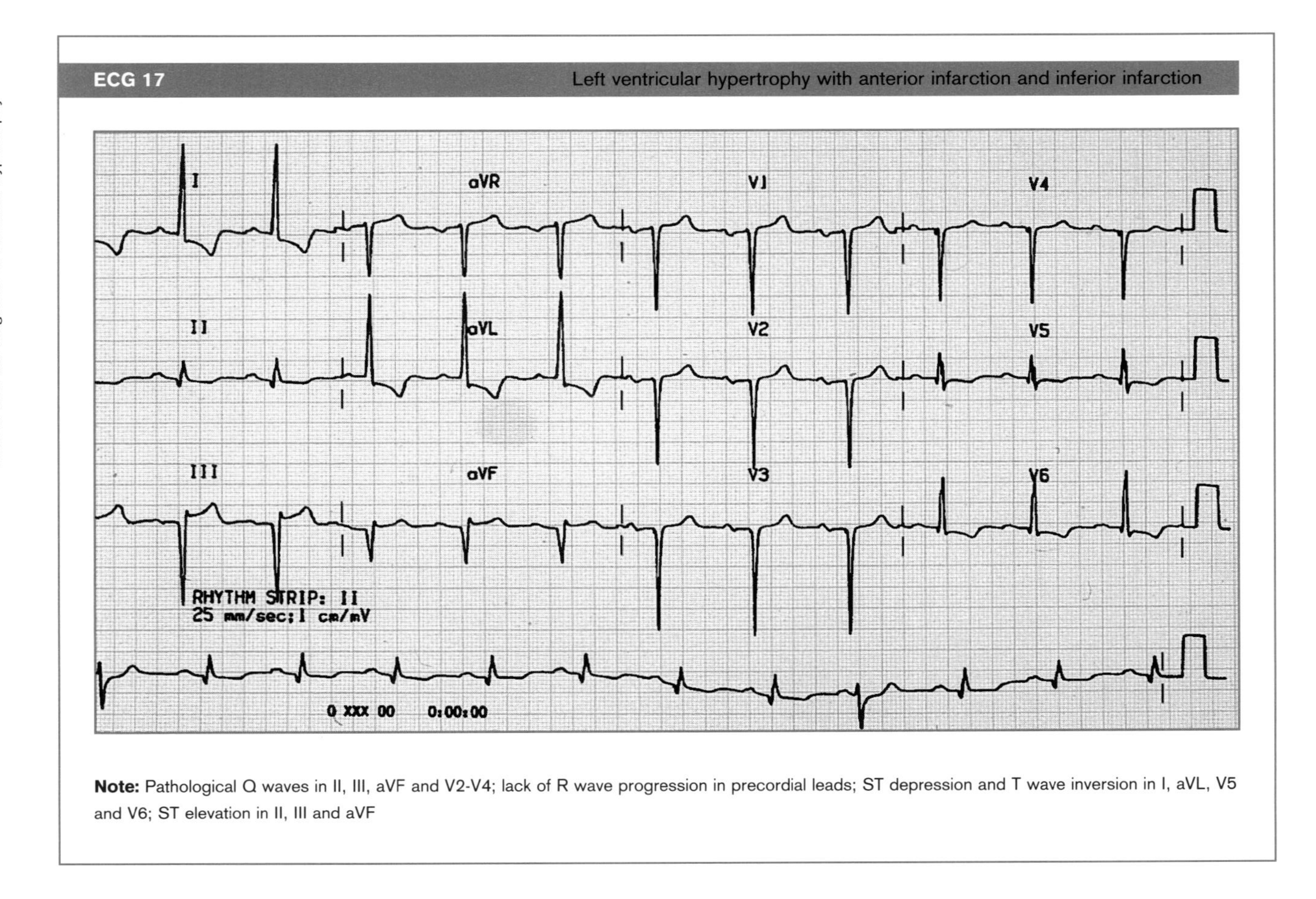

Note: Pathological Q waves in II, III, aVF and V2-V4; lack of R wave progression in precordial leads; ST depression and T wave inversion in I, aVL, V5 and V6; ST elevation in II, III and aVF

Case 18: Right ventricular hypertrophy

This ECG was recorded in a 42-year-old woman known to have had a murmur since childhood. She had recently become short of breath on exertion.

The QRS duration is increased to 120 msec. There is a secondary R wave in lead V1 (and V2) which record an rSR' complex. There are deep S waves in leads facing the left ventricle; the appearances are of right bundle branch block. The P waves in the inferior leads II, III and aVF are abnormally tall, almost reaching 5 mm in lead II. The initial positive component of the P wave in V1 (which is due to right atrial depolarisation) is also prominent. The total P wave duration is less than 120 msec - within the normal range.

Comment: This patient had an untreated ventricular septal defect with right ventricular hypertrophy. There are typical features of right atrial hypertrophy present, but very little ECG evidence of right ventricular hypertrophy. In part this is due to the fact that right bundle branch block (a frequent finding in RVH) is present and complicates the diagnosis. The ECG is often a relatively insensitive investigation in the diagnosis of RVH.

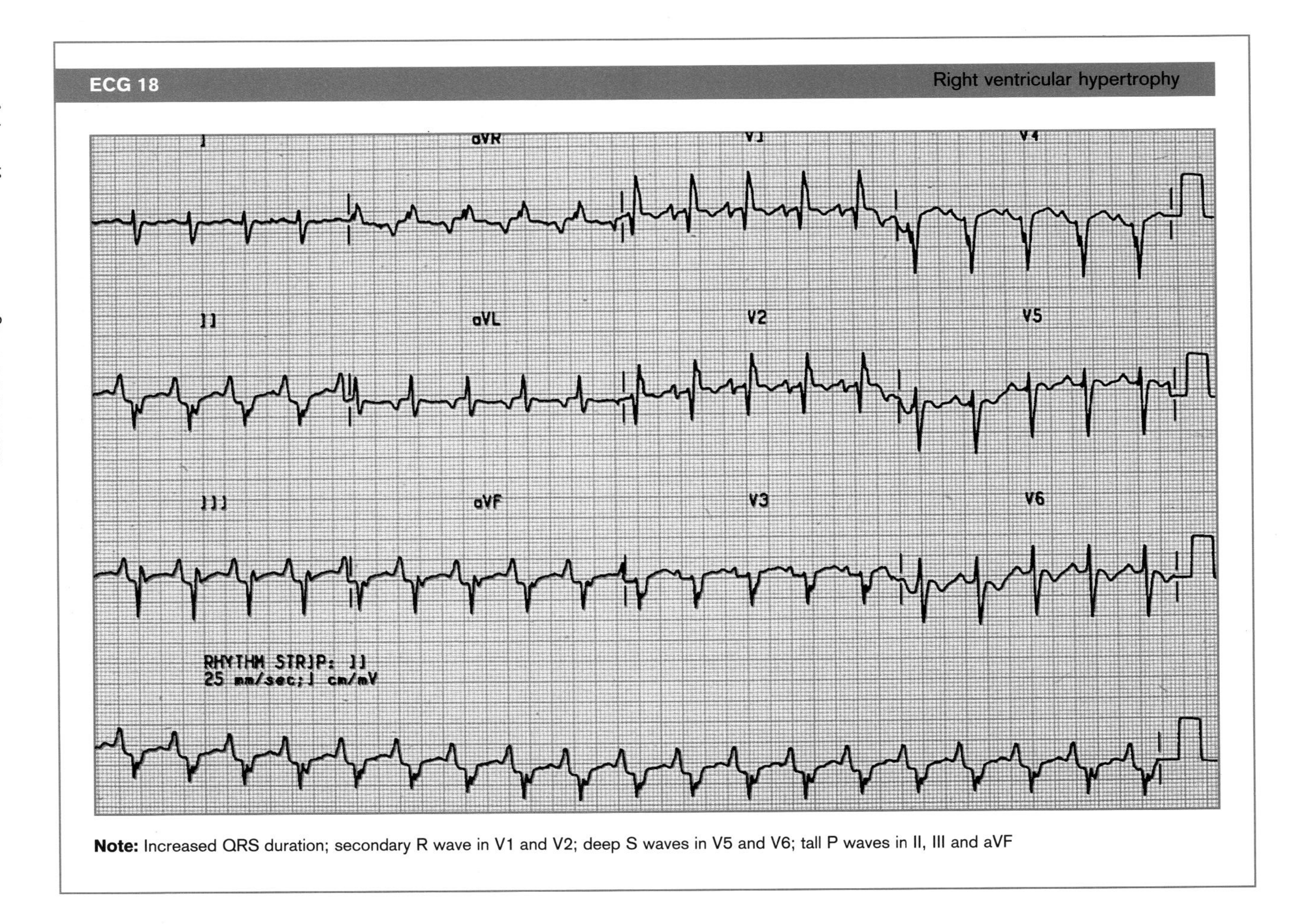

ECG 18 Right ventricular hypertrophy

Note: Increased QRS duration; secondary R wave in V1 and V2; deep S waves in V5 and V6; tall P waves in II, III and aVF

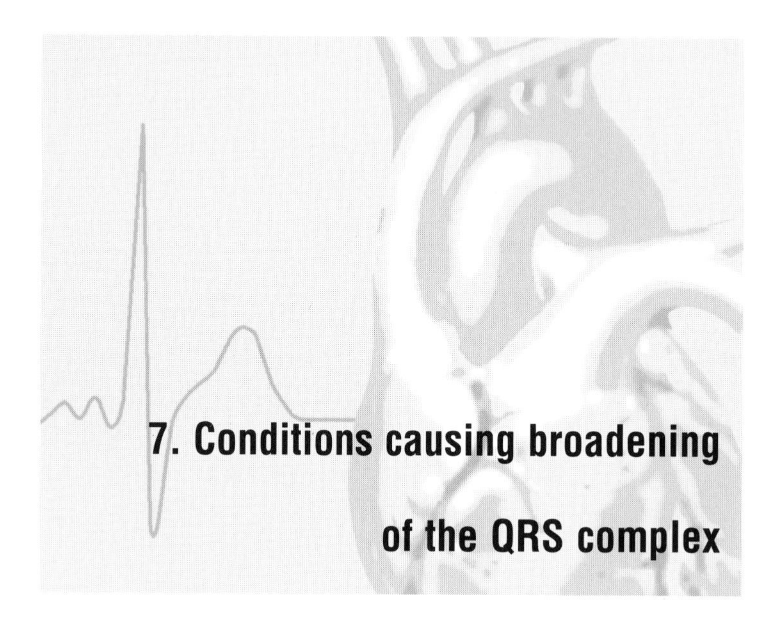

7. Conditions causing broadening of the QRS complex

Under normal circumstances the ventricles are depolarised rapidly through the specialised conducting tissue. If one or other of the bundle branches fails to conduct however, activation of the ventricle normally supplied by that bundle occurs by spread of depolarisation from the other ventricle. The delayed activation of that ventricle results in the broadening of the QRS complex beyond the upper limit of normal (100 msec).

Broadening of the QRS complex may also occur in the presence of an anomalous AV nodal bypass tract. This enables depolarisation to spread directly from the atria into ventricular myocardium, and ventricular activation commences earlier than usual because the AV node is bypassed. Ventricular depolarisation on the ECG begins prematurely with a slurred delta wave that fuses with the complex generated by normal depolarisation occurring through the AV node and conducting system. When such an ECG appearance is associated with attacks of paroxysmal supraventricular tachycardia, the condition is known as the Wolff-Parkinson-White syndrome.

Case 19: Right bundle branch block

This ECG was recorded from a 43-year-old man during an employment medical.

The QRS complexes are abnormally wide at 120 msec. There is a secondary R wave in lead V1, the complex having an rSR' appearance. There are delayed S waves in leads I, aVL, V5 and V6. Right bundle branch block (RBBB) is present.

Comment: The main ECG features of right bundle branch block are the presence of a broad QRS complex reflecting delayed ventricular depolarisation, and an M-shaped rSR' complex in V1. The initial part of ventricular depolarisation of the septum occurs normally from left to right and is recorded as an r wave in lead V1 (and q wave in V6). Left ventricular activation then occurs and a negative S wave is recorded from leads recording from the right ventricle (V1 and V2); a positive R wave is recorded from leads facing the left ventricle (V3 to V6 in this case). The last part of the ventricle to be depolarised is the right ventricular free wall, activation spreading towards V1 giving rise to the broad secondary R wave. At this time leads facing the left ventricle record an S wave. This is relatively small in this case but is prominent in Case 20.

RBBB may occur in apparently healthy individuals. It may also be seen in ischaemic disease and in conditions affecting the right ventricle. Several types of congenital heart disease are associated with RBBB.

ECG 19 Right bundle branch block

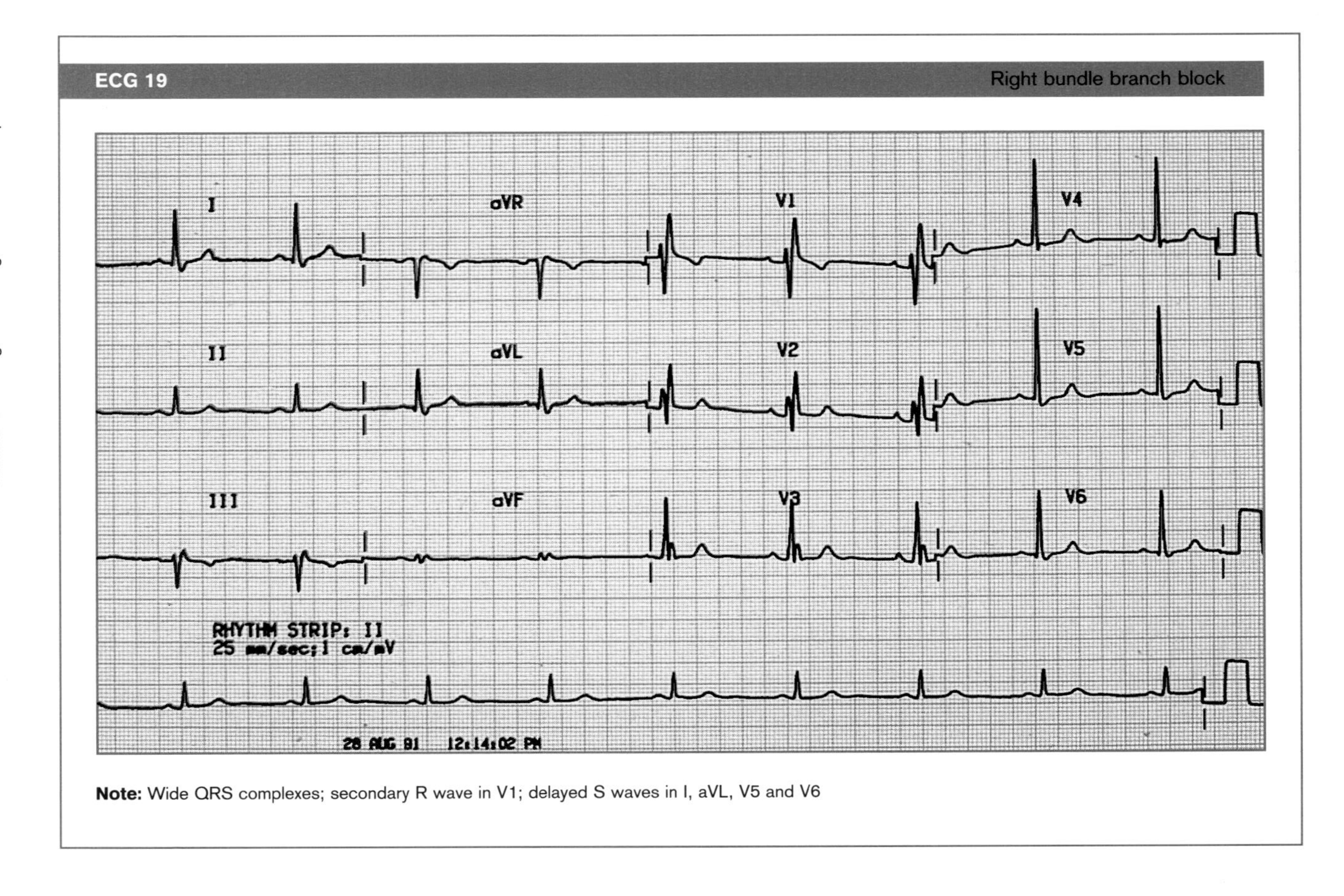

Note: Wide QRS complexes; secondary R wave in V1; delayed S waves in I, aVL, V5 and V6

Case 20: A further case of right bundle branch block

This ECG was recorded in a 48-year-old woman who developed a venous thrombosis while recovering from an operation on a fractured femur. She became acutely breathless and developed signs of right heart strain. A pulmonary embolus was subsequently confirmed.

Sinus tachycardia is present (rate 107). The QRS duration is prolonged and there is an rsR' appearance in V1 signifying the presence of RBBB. The leads overlying the right ventricle record only a small S wave (compare with the previous example). The leads recording from the lateral surface of the left ventricle show prominent S waves representing delayed right ventricular activation.

Comment: RBBB can be a feature of acute right heart strain - in this case caused by pulmonary embolism.

ECG 20

A further case of right bundle branch block

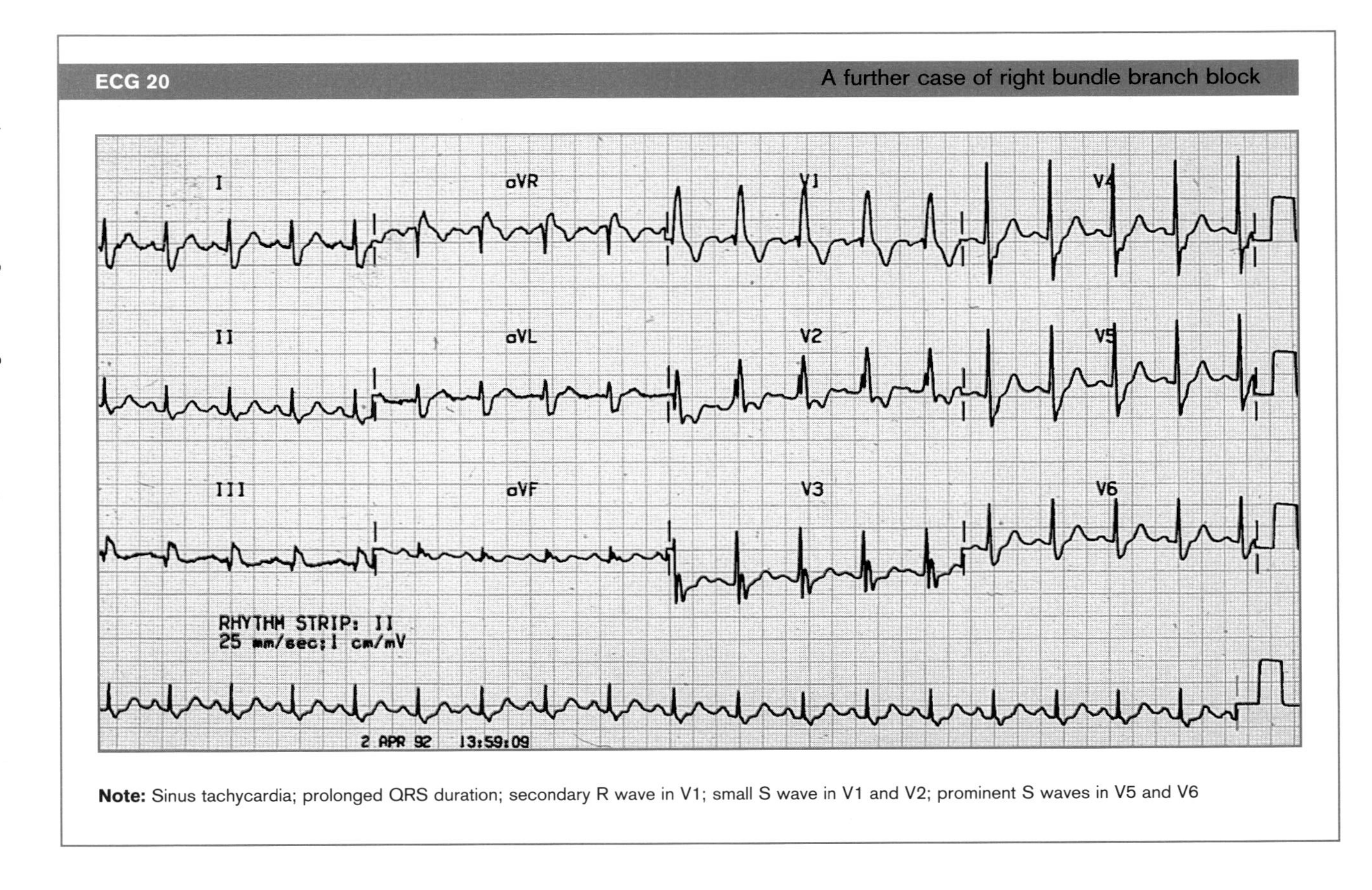

Note: Sinus tachycardia; prolonged QRS duration; secondary R wave in V1; small S wave in V1 and V2; prominent S waves in V5 and V6

Case 21: Left bundle branch block

This ECG was recorded in a 48-year-old man who had presented with a six-month history of fatigue and exertional dyspnoea. A chest X-ray had shown an enlarged heart, and echocardiography had shown diffuse impairment of ventricular function.

The QRS duration is prolonged beyond the upper limit of normal (100 msec). The q wave normally seen in V5 and V6 (resulting from septal depolarisation) is absent. There is no secondary R' wave in V1 such as occurs in right bundle branch block. These are the diagnostic features of left bundle branch block (LBBB).

Several other features that are often seen in LBBB are present in this ECG, although they are not essential to the diagnosis. The QRS complexes in leads facing the left ventricle (I, aVL, V5 and V6) show an M-shaped pattern, and there are secondary changes seen during repolarisation - ST segment depression and T wave inversion. The R waves normally seen in the precordial leads (V1 to V4) are absent. ST elevation is present in these leads and the T waves are tall. These changes must not be interpreted, however, as indicating ischaemia (or any other diagnosis) when LBBB is present.

Comment: When LBBB is present, activation of the left ventricle occurs from the right bundle branch. The interventricular septum is the first part of the ventricular myocardium to be activated, and this occurs in the opposite direction to normal, i.e. from right to left. Depolarisation of the right ventricle now occurs - directed from left to right, after which activation of the left ventricle occurs (directed from right to left). This sequence gives rise to the M-shaped appearance in leads facing the left ventricle; the initial R wave results from septal depolarisation, the negative component from right ventricular depolarisation occurring in the opposite direction, and the second R' wave from activation of the left ventricular free wall.

The most important consequence of LBBB arises from the fact that depolarisation of the AV septum at the start of ventricular activation occurs in the opposite direction to normal. None of the morphological features recorded, therefore, have the same significance as when septal depolarisation occurs normally. No deductions about the presence (or absence) of ischaemia, infarction or chamber hypertrophy should be made if the ECG shows LBBB.

ECG 21

Left bundle branch block

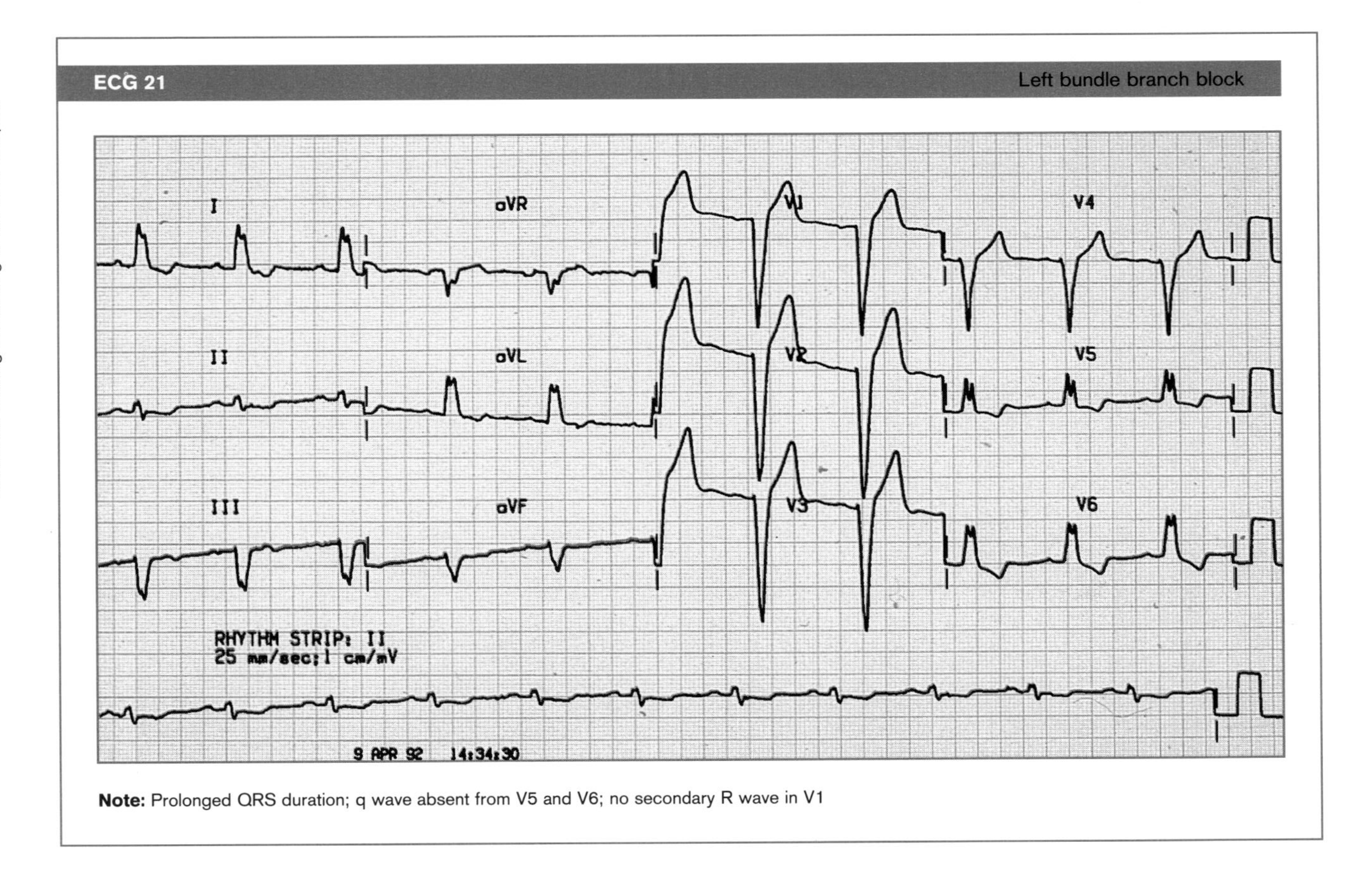

Note: Prolonged QRS duration; q wave absent from V5 and V6; no secondary R wave in V1

Left bundle branch block is nearly always associated with organic heart disease; it is seen in ischaemic disease, hypertensive heart disease and conditions diffusely involving cardiac muscle. This patient was shown to have a dilated cardiomyopathy, a condition of unknown cause that results in diffuse impairment of ventricular myocardium.

Case 22: A further case of left bundle branch block

The QRS complexes are prolonged and no q waves in leads facing the left ventricle are recorded because septal activation occurs in the opposite direction to normal. Prominent changes in the ST segment and T waves are recorded. Sinus rhythm with first-degree AV block is also present. No other diagnosis is possible from this ECG.

ECG 22

A further case of left bundle branch block

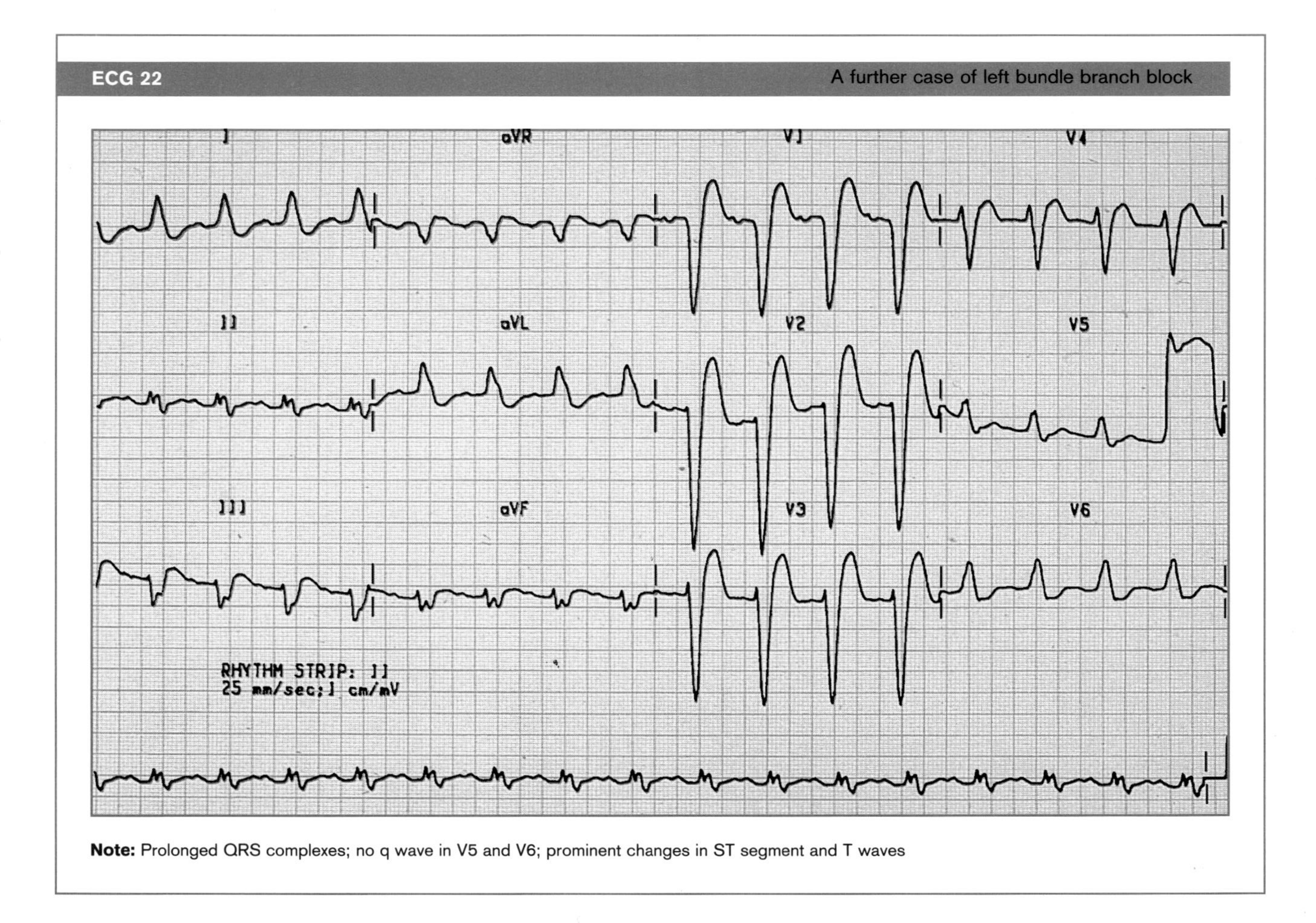

Note: Prolonged QRS complexes; no q wave in V5 and V6; prominent changes in ST segment and T waves

Case 23: The Wolff-Parkinson-White syndrome

This ECG was recorded from a 32-year-old woman with a history of recurrent attacks of supraventricular tachycardia (SVT).

The PR interval is abnormally short, i.e. less than 120 msec in duration. The total QRS duration is prolonged at 160 msec. The initial QRS deflection starts as a slurred delta wave particularly well seen in I, aVL, V5 and V6. Non-specific ST depression and T wave changes are also present.

Comment: The ECG shows the typical appearance of the Wolff-Parkinson-White (WPW) syndrome. The cardinal ECG features of this syndrome are the typical ECG changes (short PR interval and delta wave) combined with the presence of paroxysmal tachycardia.

In this condition an anomalous AV nodal bypass tract or accessory pathway is present, which provides a route through which ventricular depolarisation can occur. Ventricular depolarisation therefore occurs by a fusion of activation spreading through the anomalous bypass tract and the AV node/His-Purkinje system. The bypass tract (which consists of cardiac muscle cells) conducts the impulse more quickly than the AV node so that premature ventricular activation (pre-excitation) results. The early activation of the ventricle gives rise to the delta wave.

The ECG shows a superficial resemblance to LBBB. This occurs because the bypass tract from the atrium is connected to the upper right side of the interventricular septum - a situation analogous to LBBB where ventricular depolarisation is also initiated from the right side of the septum. For the same reasons as we have seen in LBBB, no diagnoses that rely on morphological criteria (e.g. ischaemia, infarction or hypertrophy) can be made. This type of bypass tract is sometimes known as type-B WPW syndrome.

Patients with this condition are prone to attacks of supraventricular tachycardia because under certain conditions the bypass tract enables a circuit to be established, whereby activation of both atria and ventricles occurs repetitively through a circus movement of depolarisation passing from the ventricles retrogradely to the atria via the bypass tract, only to be conducted anterogradely back to the ventricles through the AV node.

ECG 23 The Wolff-Parkinson-White syndrome

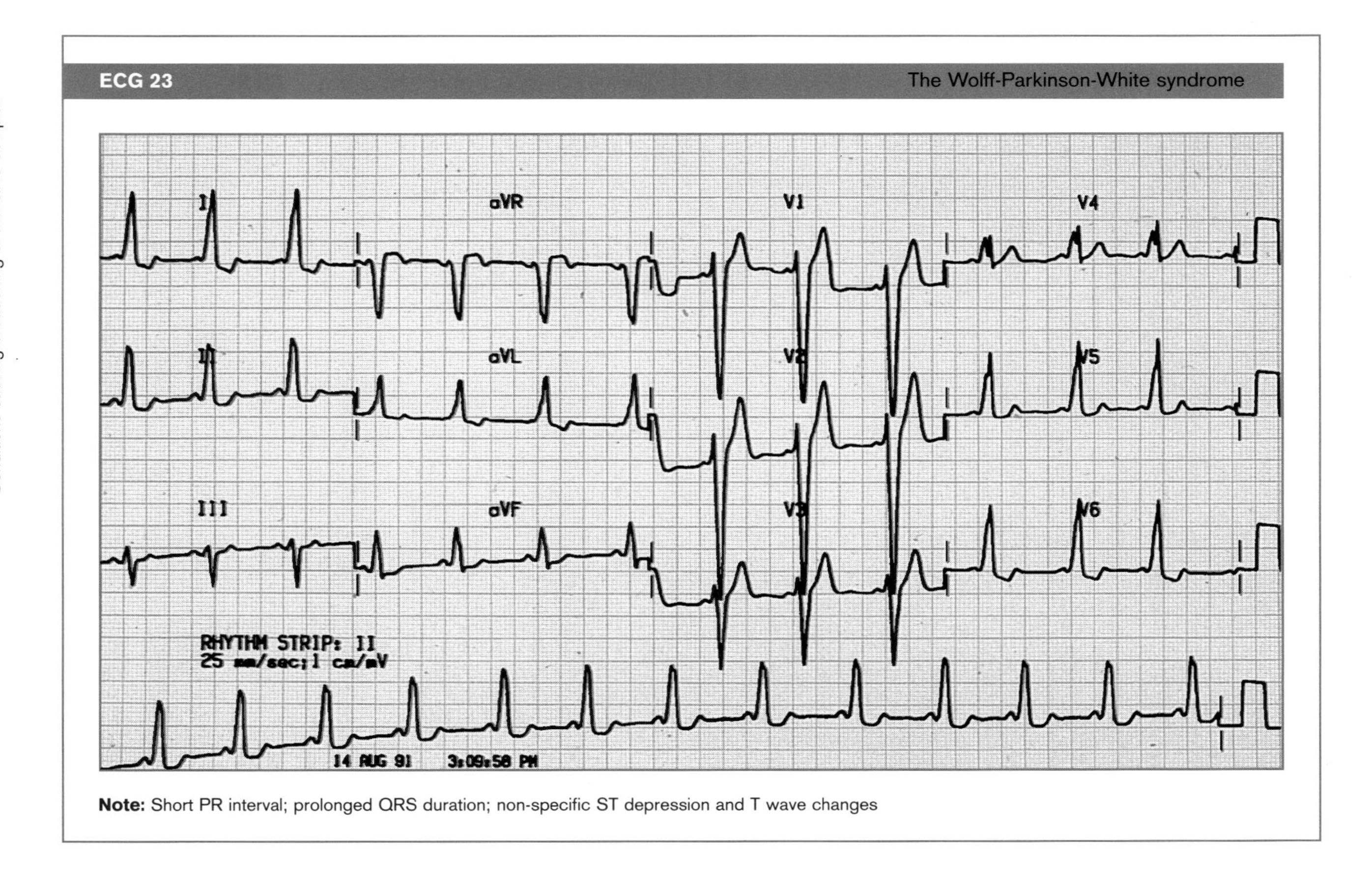

Note: Short PR interval; prolonged QRS duration; non-specific ST depression and T wave changes

Case 24: Wolff-Parkinson-White syndrome type-A

This ECG has a superficial resemblance to RBBB because in this case the bypass tract causes premature activation of the left ventricle and ventricular depolarisation occurs in a similar sequence to RBBB.

ECG 24

Wolff-Parkinson-White syndrome type-A

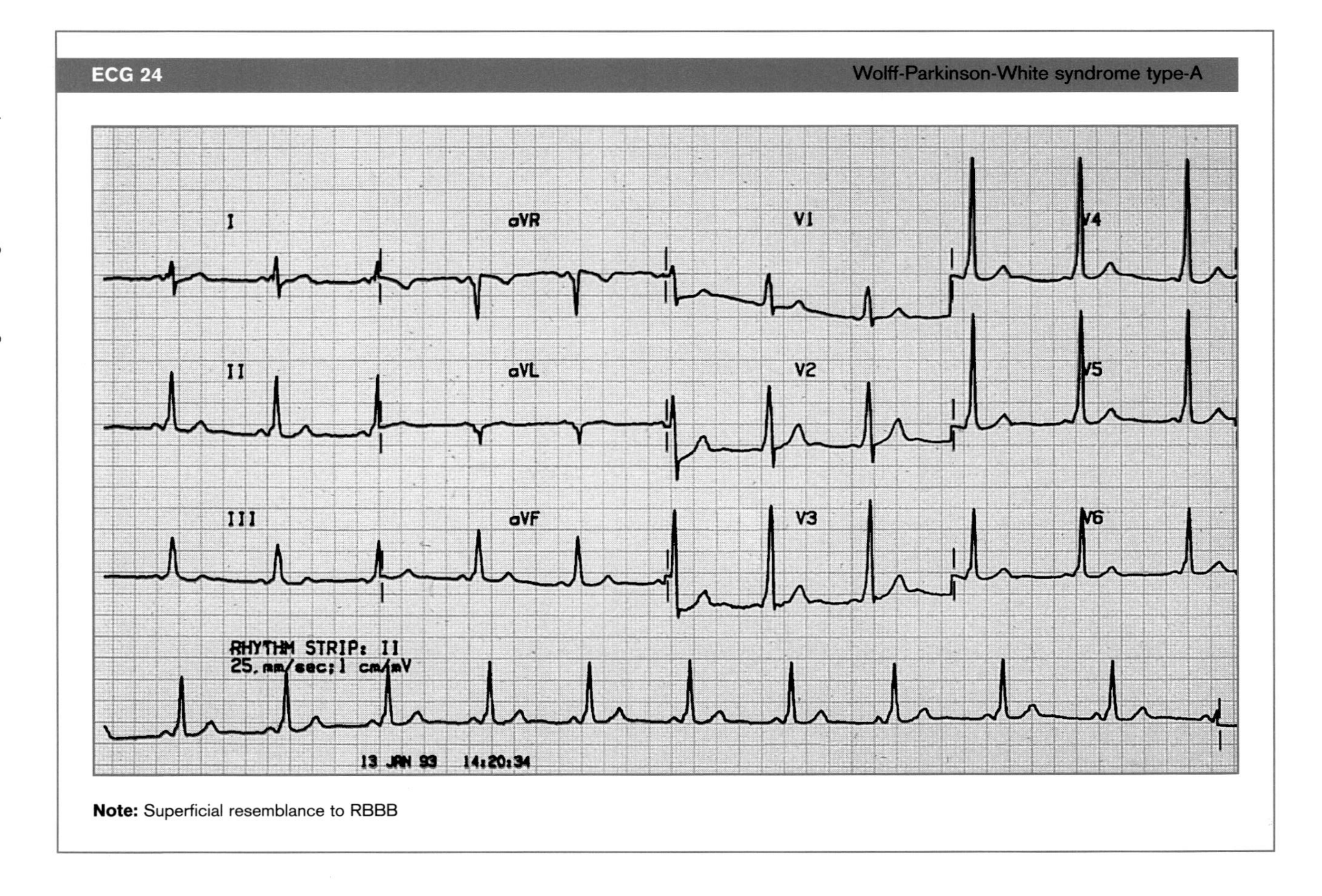

Note: Superficial resemblance to RBBB

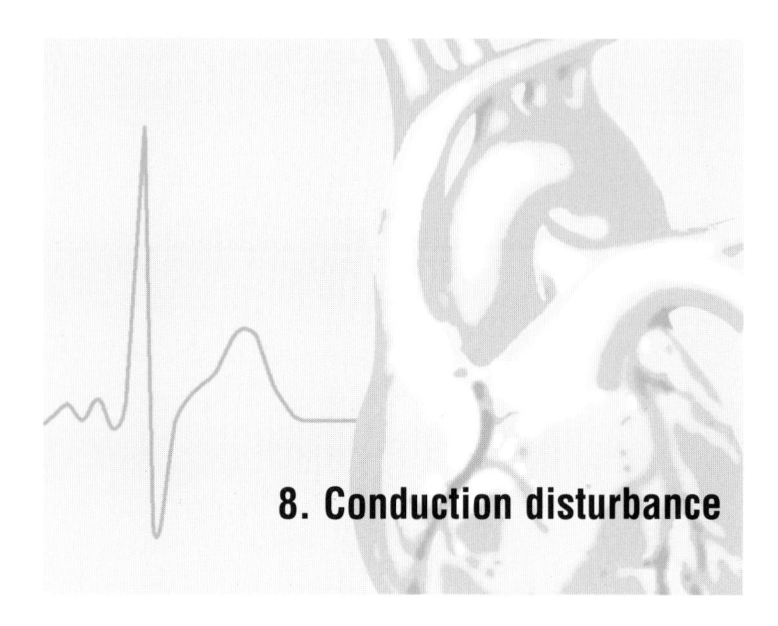

8. Conduction disturbance

The final section of this book (Chapters 8 to 10) is devoted to illustrations of common arrhythmias and disorders of impulse conduction. A normal cardiac rate is defined arbitrarily as lying between 60 and 100 beats per minute. Below a rate of 60 bradycardia is present, while rates above 100 are termed tachycardia. This definition does not take account of the fact that the rate may be entirely normal, yet the origin of the rhythm may be abnormal. Similarly, an entirely normal cardiac rhythm may have a rate outside these limits depending on the physiological requirements of the individual.

The generation or propagation of the cardiac action potential may be disturbed at any site between its origin in the sinoatrial node and the more distal conduction pathways. The following examples illustrate some of the common patterns encountered.

ECG 25: Sinus bradycardia

Sinus rhythm at a rate of 46 per minute is present. This is usually an entirely normal rhythm, and is common in fit individuals.

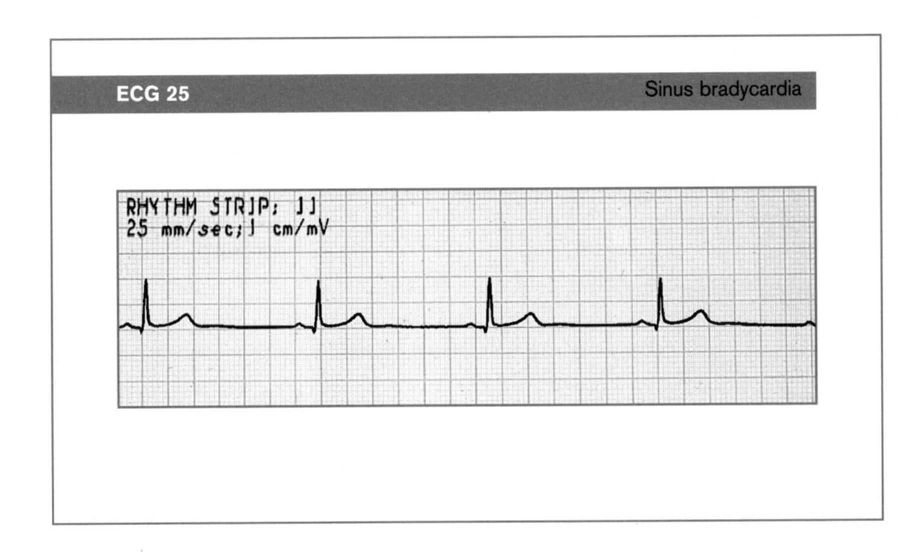

ECG 26: Sinoatrial block

The sinus node depolarises normally, but there is intermittent failure of conduction of the impulse to the atrial myocardium (exit block) with consequent failure of atrial depolarisation. The subsequent discharge from the SA node triggers atrial depolarisation at the normal time, so the pause resulting from the missed beat is double the basic cycle length. With more prolonged episodes of block, prolonged pauses will result if no escape rhythm from a subsidiary pacemaker supervenes - **ECG 27**.

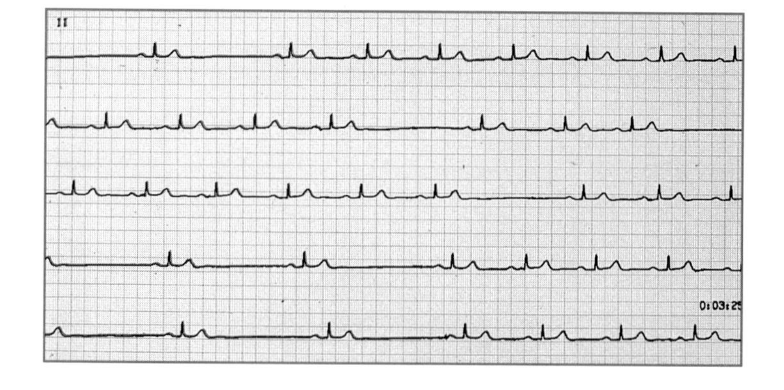

ECG 27 — Sinoatrial block

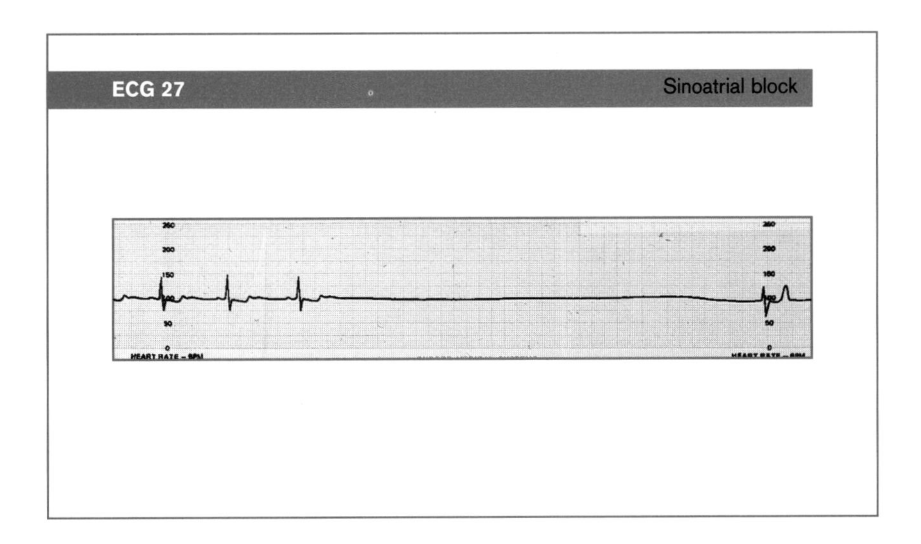

ECG 28-30: Atrioventricular block

Atrioventricular (AV) block exists when conduction delay occurs at the AV junction. It is not possible from the surface ECG to say whether the site of the block is in the AV node or bundle of His. Three degrees of AV block are recognised.

First-degree AV block

ECG 28: The PR interval is consistently prolonged but every beat is conducted to the ventricles.

Second-degree AV block

Intermittent failure of conduction occurs so that some atrial complexes are not conducted to the ventricles. The ECG shows some P waves that are not followed by QRS complexes. Two types of second-degree block are recognised:

Mobitz type-1 (Wenckebach): Increasing conduction delay occurs with successive beats until failure of AV conduction occurs. **ECG 29** shows P waves followed by QRS complexes, but the PR interval increases progressively as the degree of block increases with successive beats. Failure of conduction ultimately occurs and the ECG shows a P wave that is not followed by a QRS complex. During the pause that arises from the dropped beat, the AV junction recovers and the next sinus beat is conducted to the ventricles. The cycle is often repeated.

Mobitz type-2: In this condition intermittent failure of AV conduction occurs. The PR interval may be normal or prolonged, but it is constant. The failure of AV conduction results in P waves occurring at the expected time that are not followed by QRS complexes. In the example **ECG 30** there is failure to conduct alternate beats; 2:1 AV block is an alternative description.

ECG 28 First-degree AV block

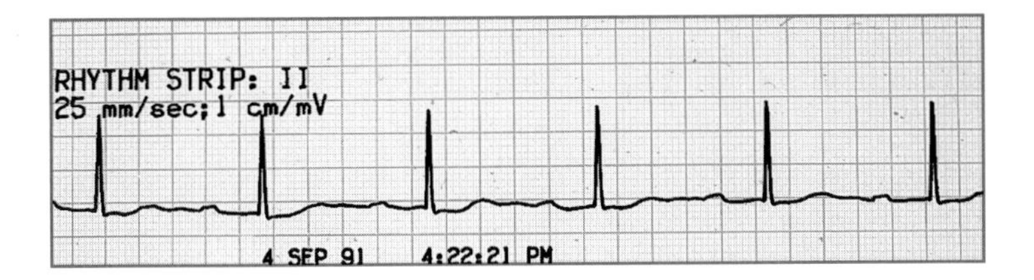

ECG 29 Second-degree AV block, Mobitz type-1 (Wenckebach)

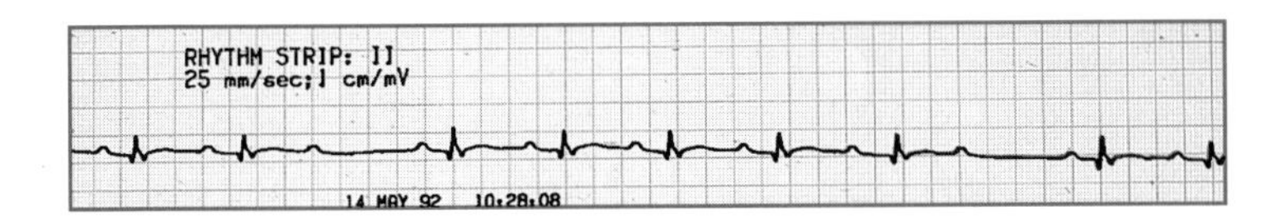

ECG 30 Second-degree AV block, Mobitz type-2

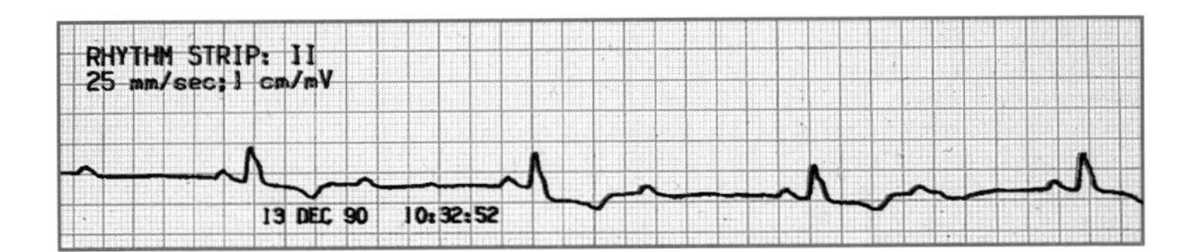

ECG 31-33: Atrioventricular block

Third-degree (complete) AV block

Complete failure of AV conduction is present, and no electrical activity is conducted from atria to ventricles. When sinus rhythm is present the ECG will show P waves but these do not trigger ventricular depolarisation, which is maintained by an escape rhythm initiated from a separate subsidiary pacemaker situated in the AV junction, conducting system or ventricular myocardium. Depolarisation of the atria and ventricles occurs independently and there is no discernible relationship between the P waves and the QRS complexes on the ECG - **ECG 31, ECG 32**. Failure of the escape rhythm will result in ventricular asystole and cardiac arrest unless an escape rhythm becomes re-established - **ECG 33**.

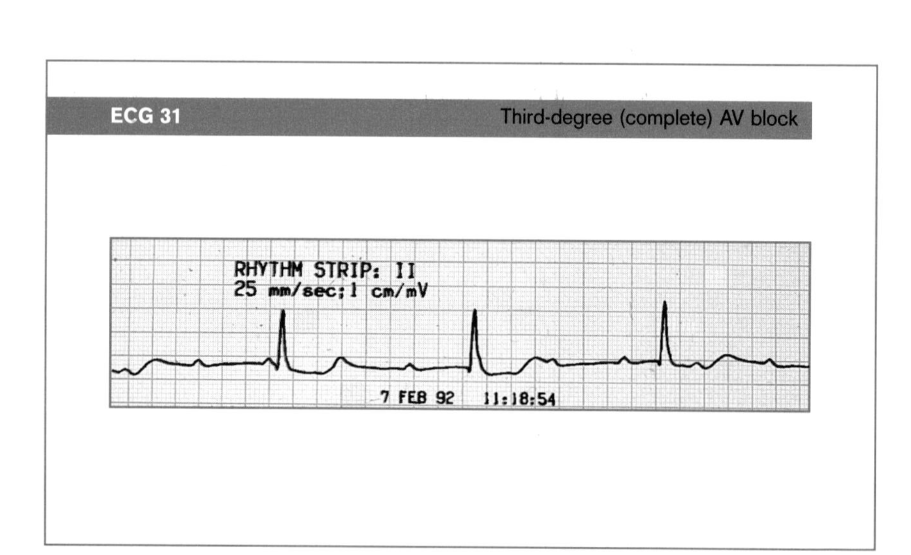

ECG 32 Third-degree (complete) AV block

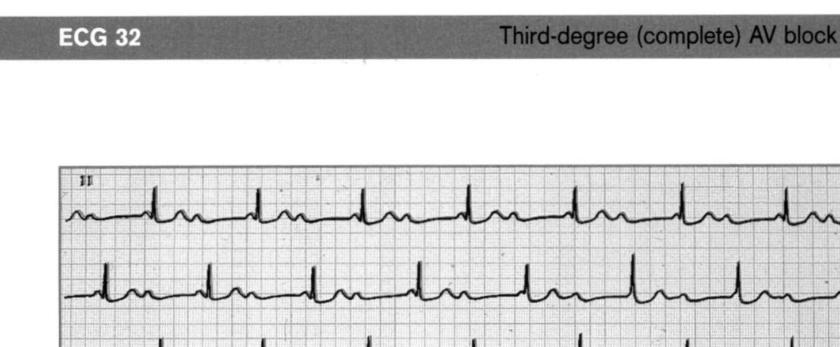

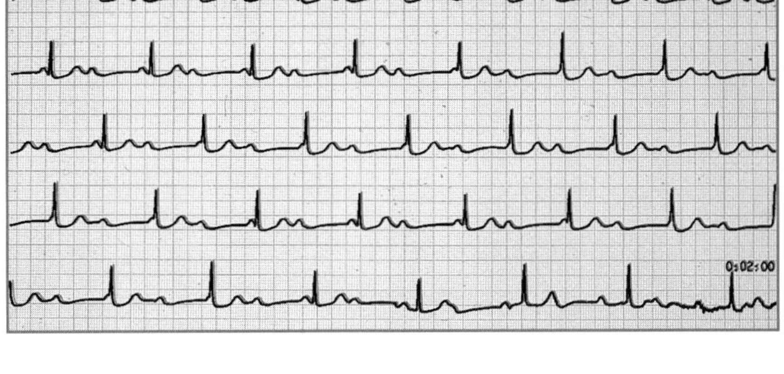

ECG 33 Third-degree (complete) AV block

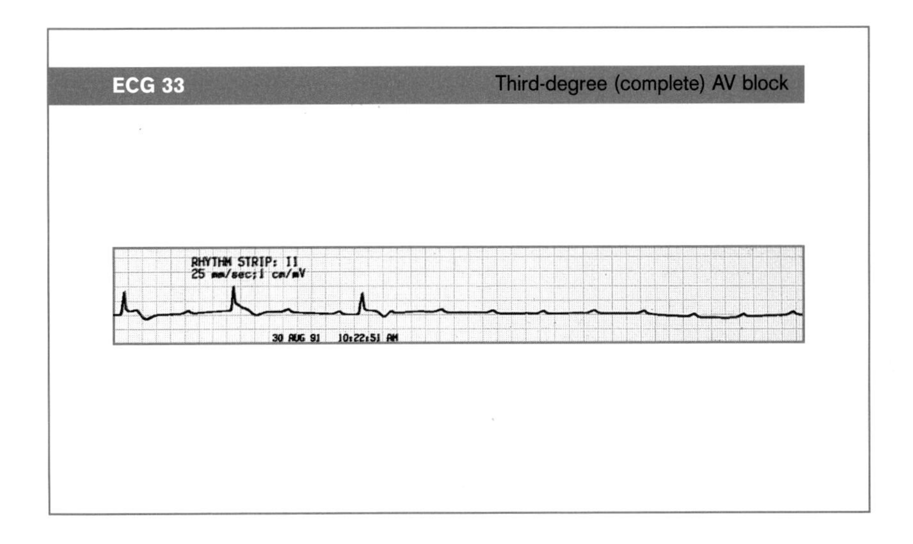

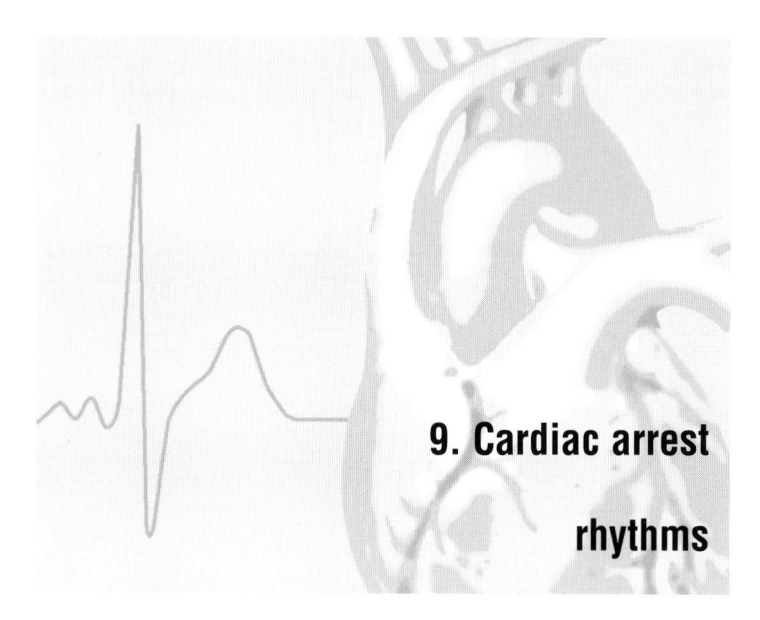

9. Cardiac arrest rhythms

ECG 34-36: Ventricular fibrillation

ECG 34: In ventricular fibrillation all co-ordinated electrical activity is lost, and the ECG shows a series of bizarre irregular complexes of random frequency and amplitude. Co-ordinated ventricular contraction ceases and cardiac arrest results. The amplitude of the complexes in ventricular fibrillation decreases with time (**ECG 35, ECG 36**) until asystole supervenes. Defibrillation becomes progressively more difficult the longer it is delayed.

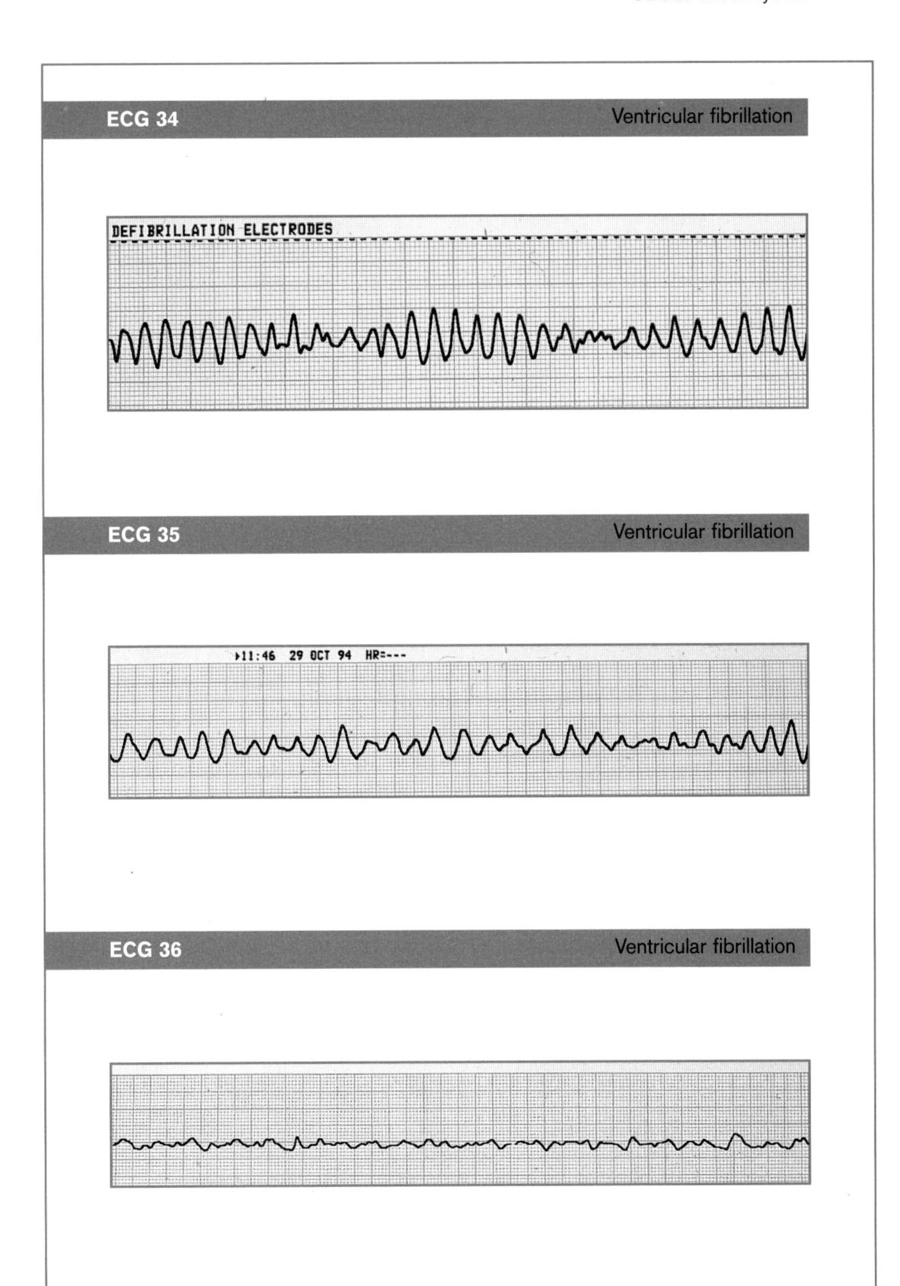

ECG 34 Ventricular fibrillation

ECG 35 Ventricular fibrillation

ECG 36 Ventricular fibrillation

ECG 37: Asystole

No electrical activity from the heart is recorded on the ECG. Some baseline drift or artifact caused by ventilation or cardiopulmonary resuscitation is usually present; a completely straight line usually means that an ECG lead has become detached.

ECG 38: Asystole with persistent P waves

Complete AV block with no escape rhythm exists; P waves may persist briefly at the onset of ventricular asystole. If no ventricular escape rhythm becomes established all electrical activity is ultimately lost.

Electromechanical dissociation

This is not an electrocardiographic diagnosis, but is mentioned here for completeness. Electromechanical dissociation (EMD) is the term used to describe the clinical picture of cardiac arrest with an ECG rhythm that would be expected to produce a cardiac output. The ECG is often normal or nearly normal.

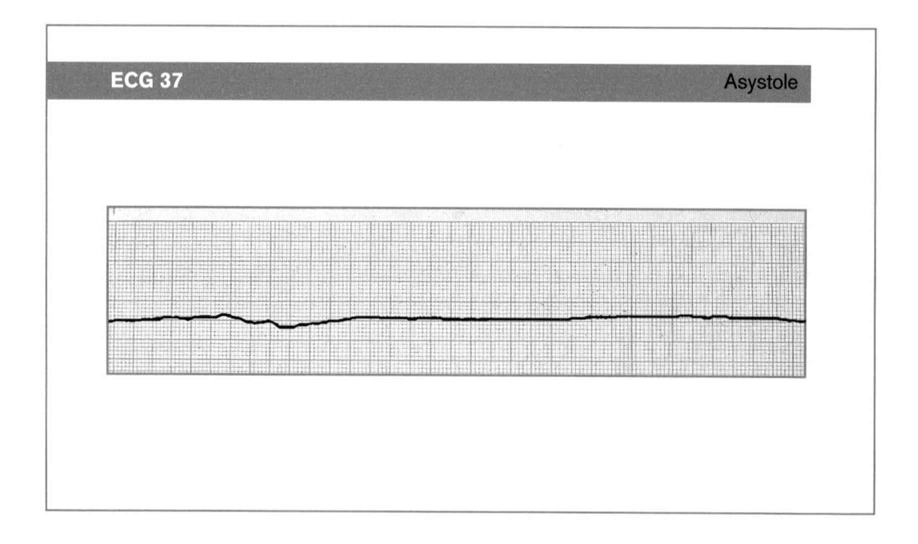

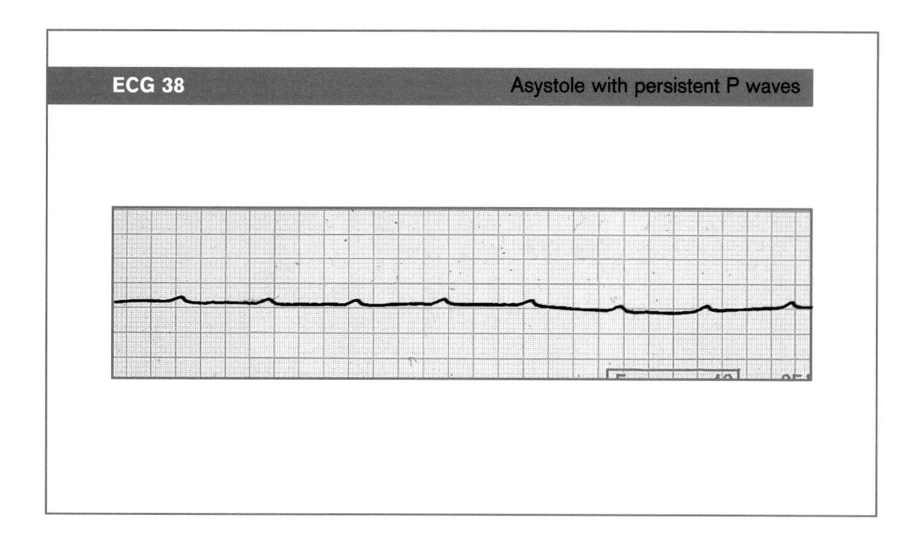

ECG 38 Asystole with persistent P waves

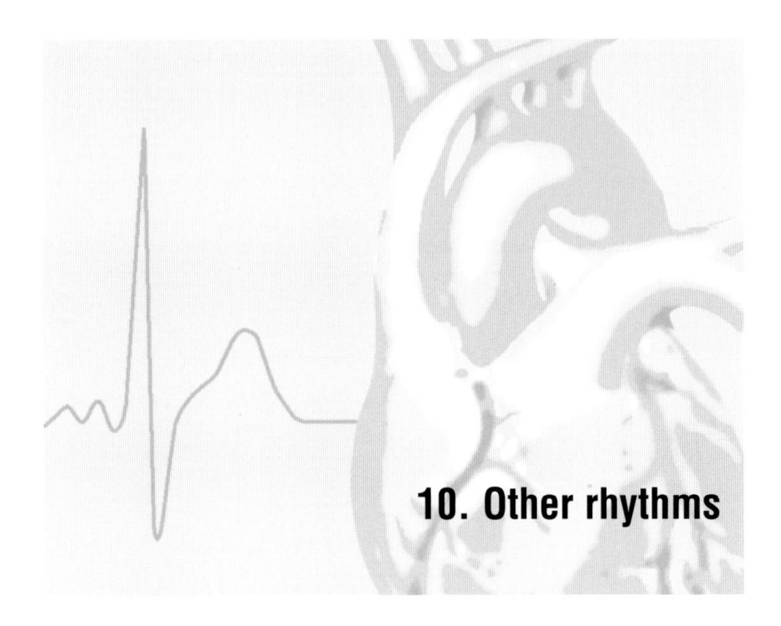

10. Other rhythms

In this chapter some cardiac rhythms other than sinus rhythm are illustrated.

ECG 39-41 Atrial fibrillation

This is the most common arrhythmia encountered in clinical practice. The process of atrial depolarisation is unco-ordinated and appears to occur in a random chaotic fashion. It is recognised on the ECG by the lack of P waves or any other evidence of co-ordinated atrial depolarisation. Random disorganised atrial electrical activity, best seen in leads V1 and V2, is usually present - **ECG 39**. Ventricular depolarisation occurs irregularly, and the rate of ventricular response will depend on conditions in the AV node. Very fast rates of conduction are possible - **ECG 39A**, and may produce heart failure.

ECG 39 Atrial fibrillation

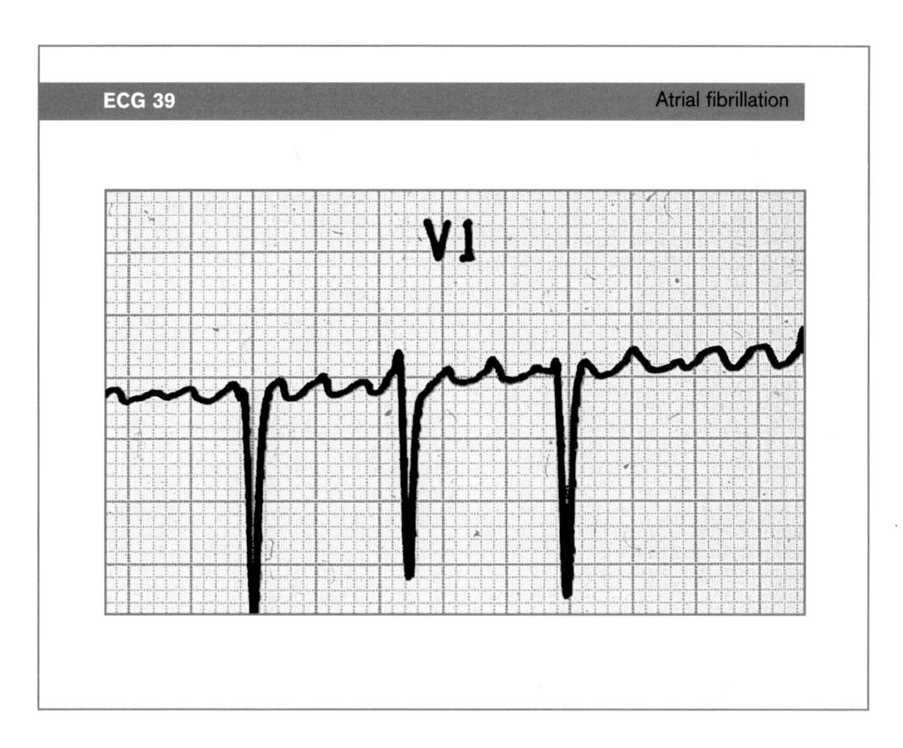

ECG 39A Atrial fibrillation

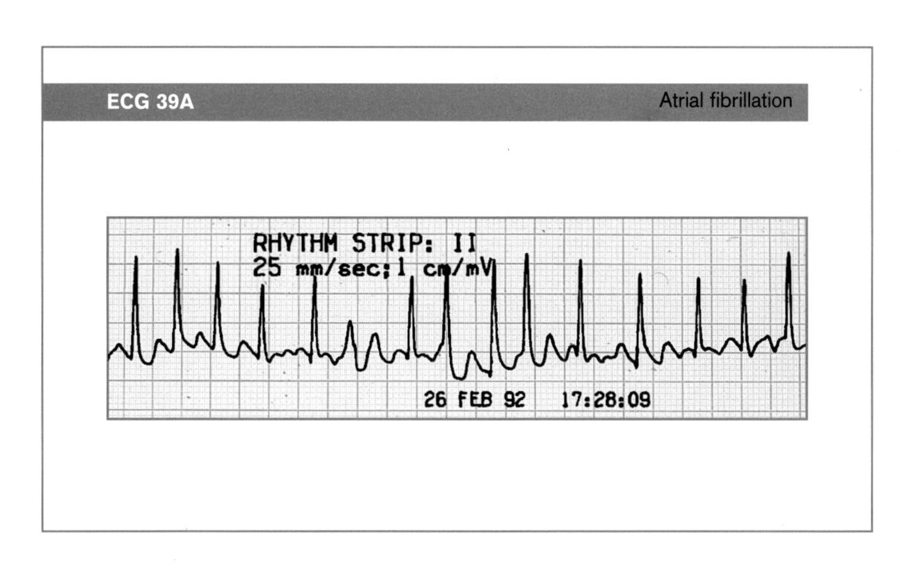

Block in conduction at the AV node (either inherent or produced by drugs such as digoxin, verapamil or beta-blockers) will slow the rate of ventricular response - **ECG 40**. Should complete heart block be present the ventricles are depolarised from a subsidiary pacemaker usually in the AV junction or ventricular myocardium, and the ventricular rhythm will usually be regular. **ECG 41** shows this, and demonstrates the irregular atrial activity.

ECG 40 — Atrial fibrillation

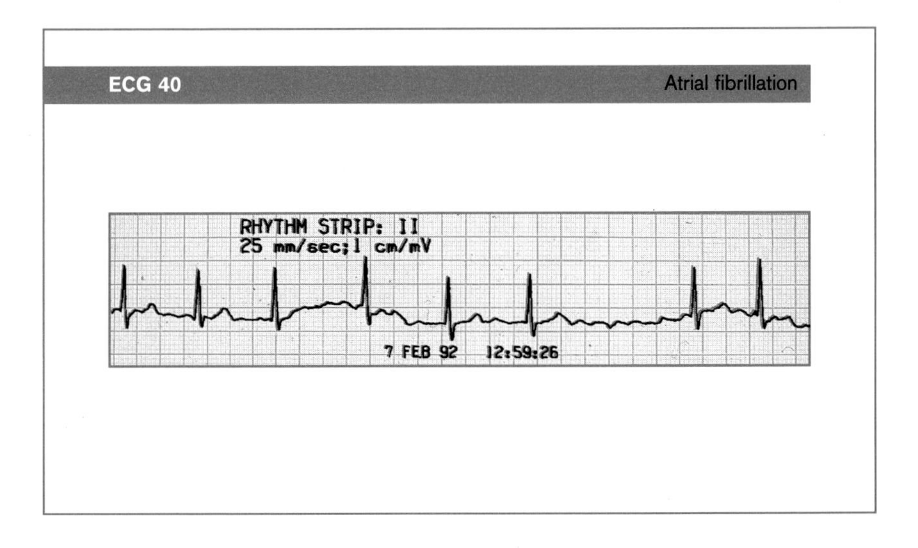

ECG 41 — Atrial fibrillation

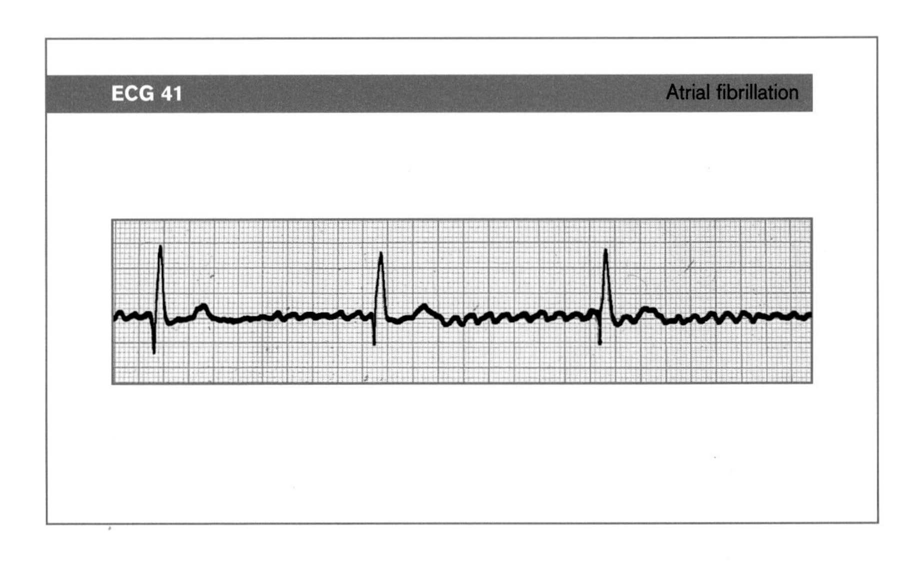

ECG 42-43: Atrial flutter

Atrial flutter is a type of atrial tachycardia in which atrial depolarisation occurs at a rapid rate (usually around 300 per minute). The rhythm is thought to arise from a re-entrant tachycardia that is propagated within the atria. Atrial activity is represented on the ECG as a series of regular sawtooth waves usually best seen in the inferior leads - **ECG 42**. The rate of ventricular response will depend on the degree of AV block present, and an irregular rhythm often results. **ECG 43** shows variable AV block in response to atrial flutter; left ventricular hypertrophy is also present.

ECG 42 Atrial flutter

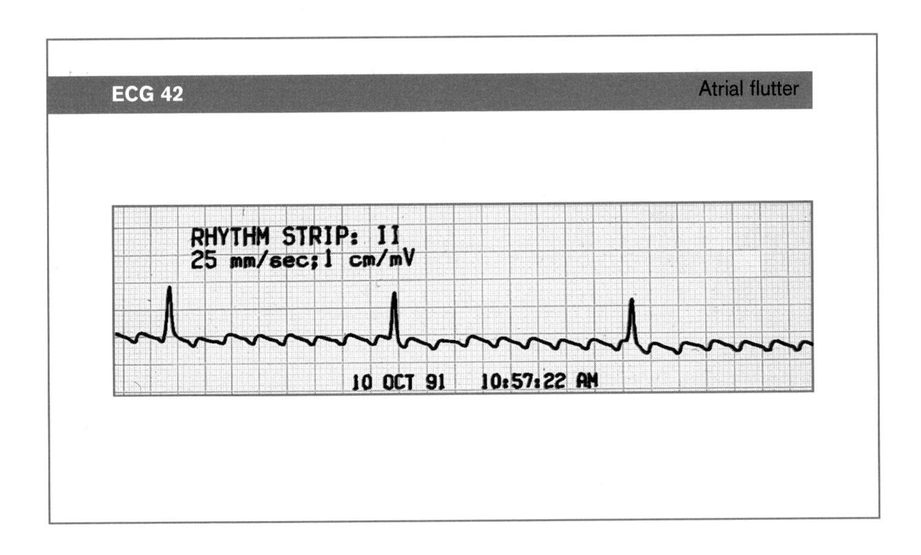

ECG 43 Atrial flutter

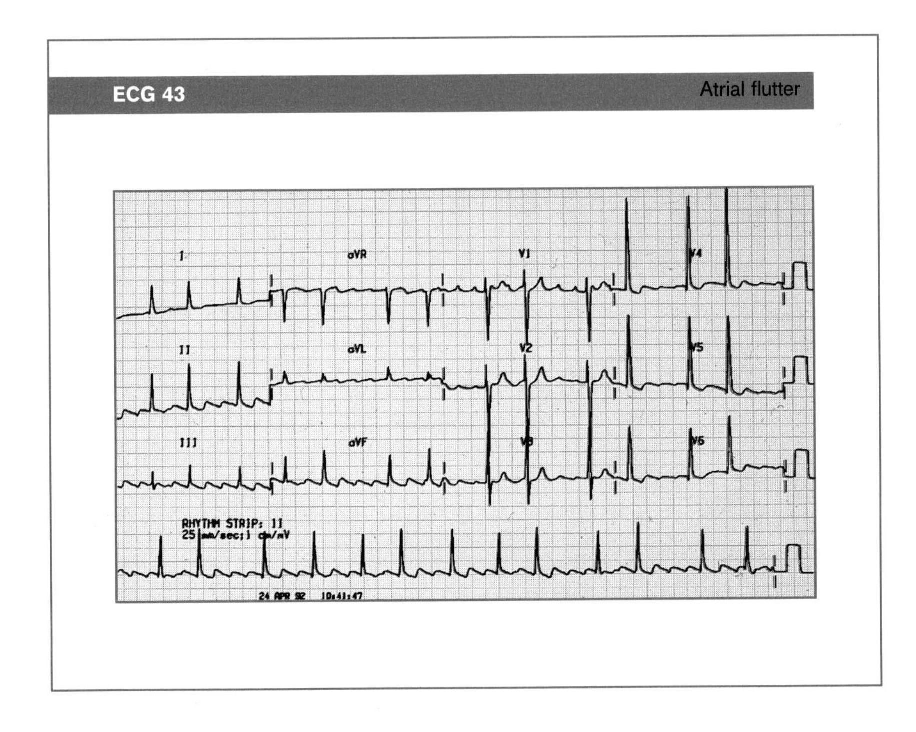

ECG 44-46: Junctional rhythms

When ventricular depolarisation is initiated within the AV junction (the AV node and bundle of His) a junctional rhythm results. This may occur because the normal supraventricular rhythm fails, for example if sinoatrial block occurs, or because the AV node fails to conduct atrial depolarisation to the ventricles. In the former situation P waves will be absent - **ECG 44, ECG 45**, unless retrograde conduction of ventricular depolarisation through the AV node into the atria occurs. In this case a P′ wave will be recorded during retrograde activation of the atria. In **ECG 46** a P′ wave is seen before the QRS complex; it is inverted in the inferior leads, suggesting that atrial depolarisation is occurring in the opposite direction to the normal manner seen in sinus rhythm. In some cases, the P′ wave may follow the QRS complex and distort the T wave.

A junctional escape rhythm may maintain cardiac output when complete AV block is present (see **ECG 31**).

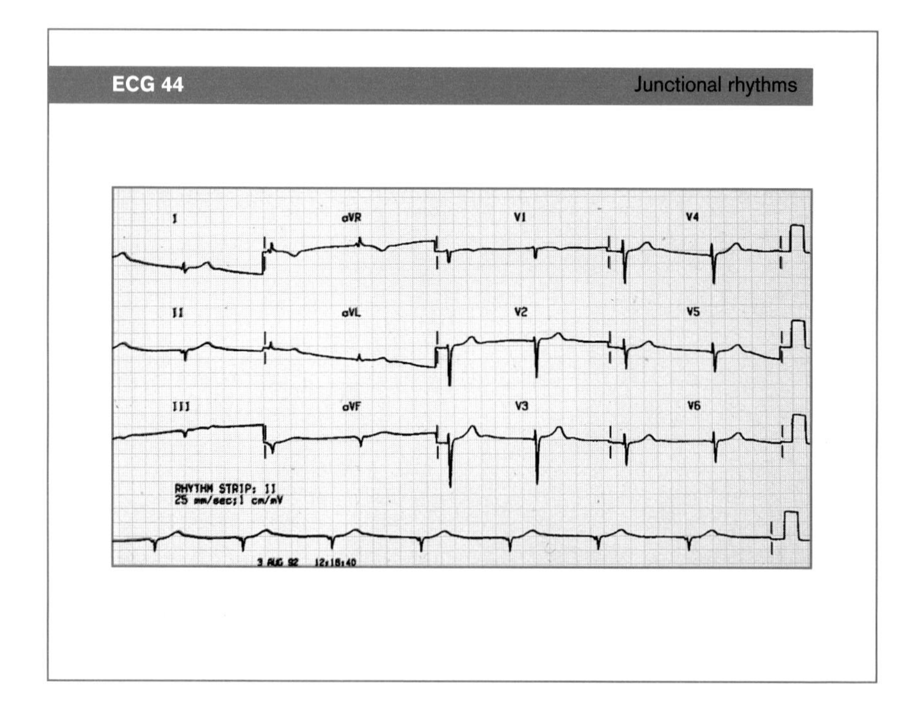

ECG 44 Junctional rhythms

ECG 45 — Junctional rhythms

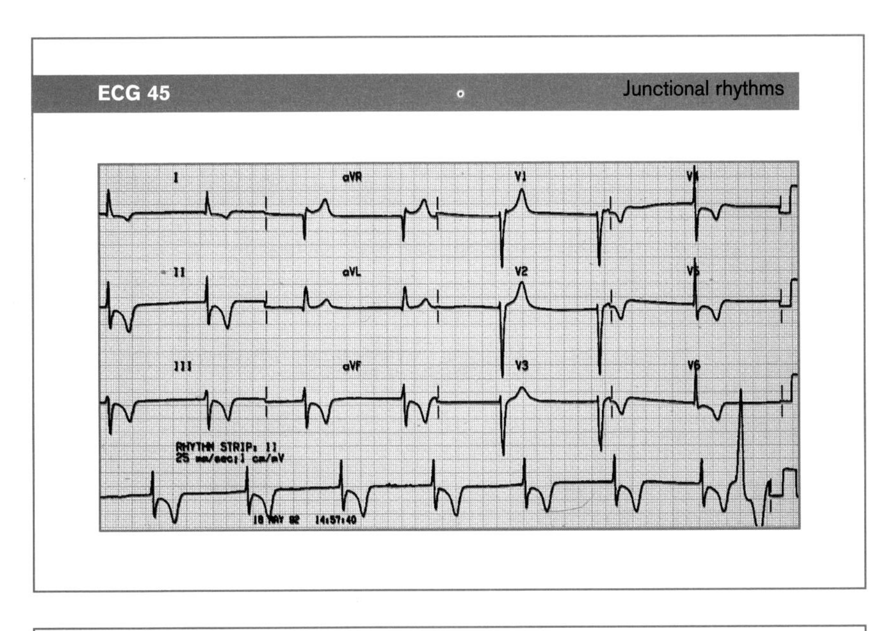

ECG 46 — Junctional rhythms

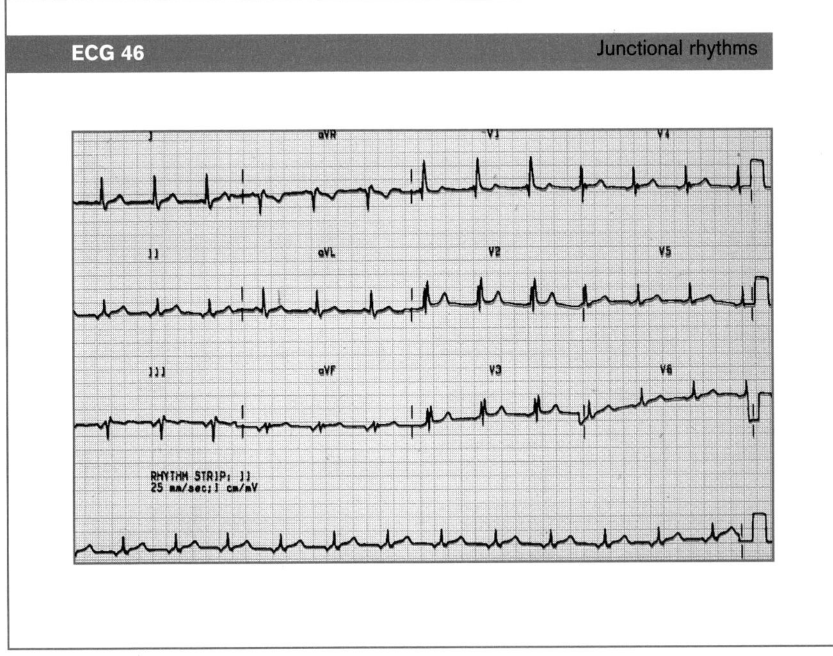

ECG 47-49: Ectopic beats

Ectopic beats arise from an ectopic focus within the atrial or ventricular myocardium or conducting tissue. If occurring before the next anticipated beat they are known as premature beats, while if occurring late, after a pause in the basic rhythm, they are known as escape beats.

Atrial premature beats

ECG 47: Every sinus beat is followed by a premature beat. The QRS morphology of the sinus and premature beats is the same. P' waves can be seen distorting the T waves of the sinus QRS complexes - compare the T waves of the ectopic beat with that of the preceding sinus beat.

ECG 47 Atrial premature beats

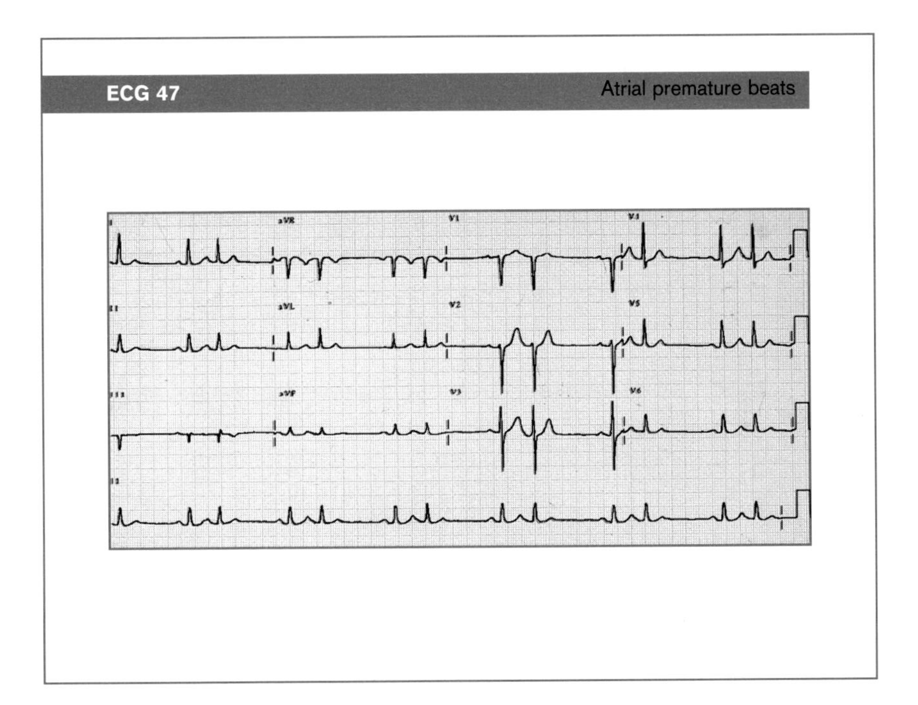

Ventricular premature beats

ECG 48: Every sinus beat is conducted normally giving rise to a narrow QRS complex. After every sinus beat a ventricular premature beat is seen as a broad complex beat. When ventricular premature beats alternate with normal sinus beats in this fashion ventricular bigeminy is said to be present. When ectopic beats arise from several foci, multifocal ventricular premature beats are said to be present - **ECG 49.**

ECG 48 Ventricular premature beats

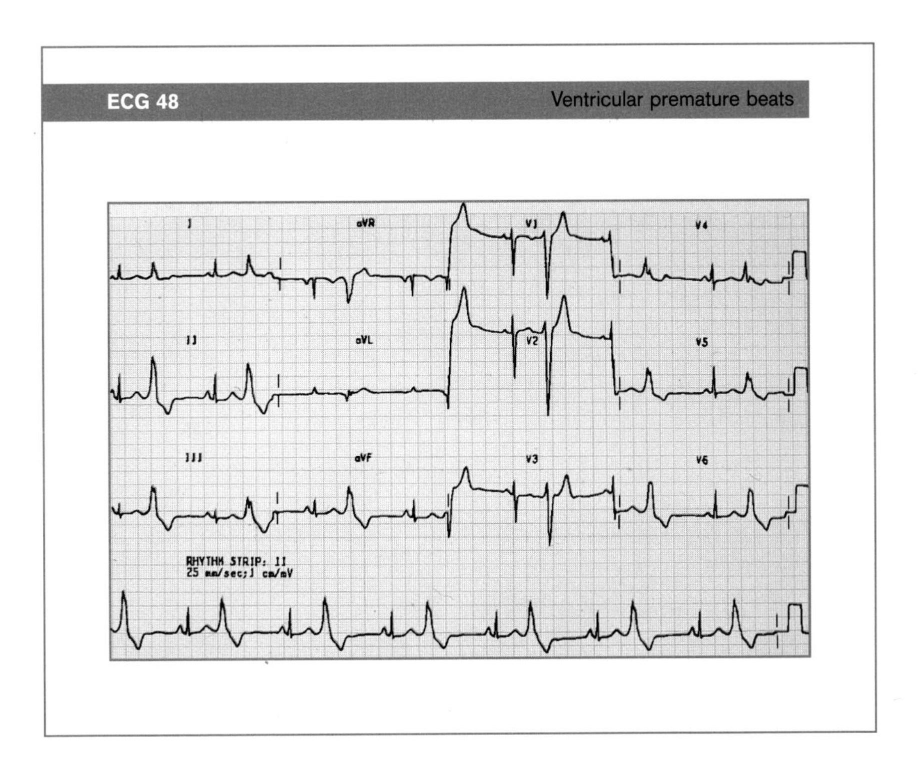

ECG 49 Ventricular premature beats

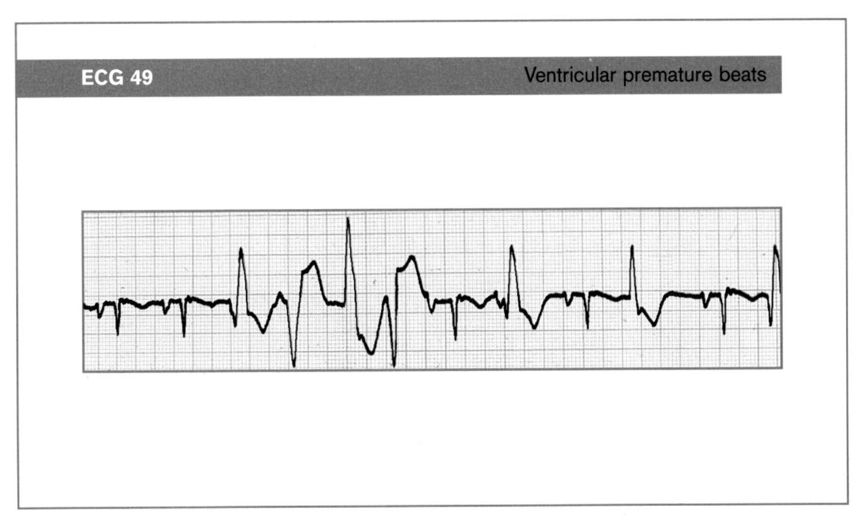

ECG 50-51: Supraventricular tachycardia

Most cases of supraventricular tachycardia (SVT) arise from the AV junction and the term junctional tachycardia is then more correct. In most cases the tachycardia is maintained by a circuit involving the AV node and an AV nodal bypass tract. The bypass tract may be situated within the AV node itself, when the tachycardia is described as an atrioventricular nodal re-entrant tachycardia (or AVNRT). When there is a direct connection between atrial and ventricular myocardium outside the AV node (as in the Wolff-Parkinson-White syndrome) the term atrioventricular re-entrant tachycardia (AVRT) is used. Differentiation between the two is often impossible from the surface ECG.

ECG 50: SVT recorded in V1.

ECG 51: SVT recorded in V6.

ECG 50 Supraventricular tachycardia

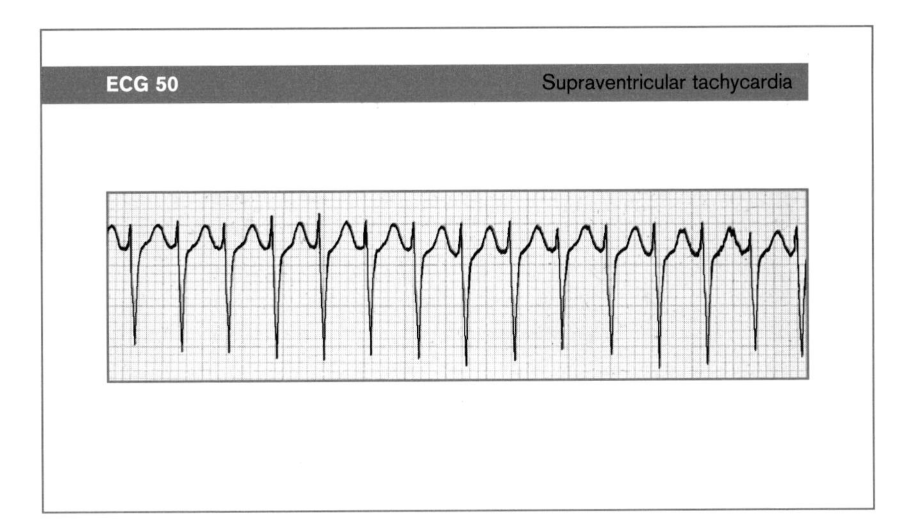

ECG 51 Supraventricular tachycardia

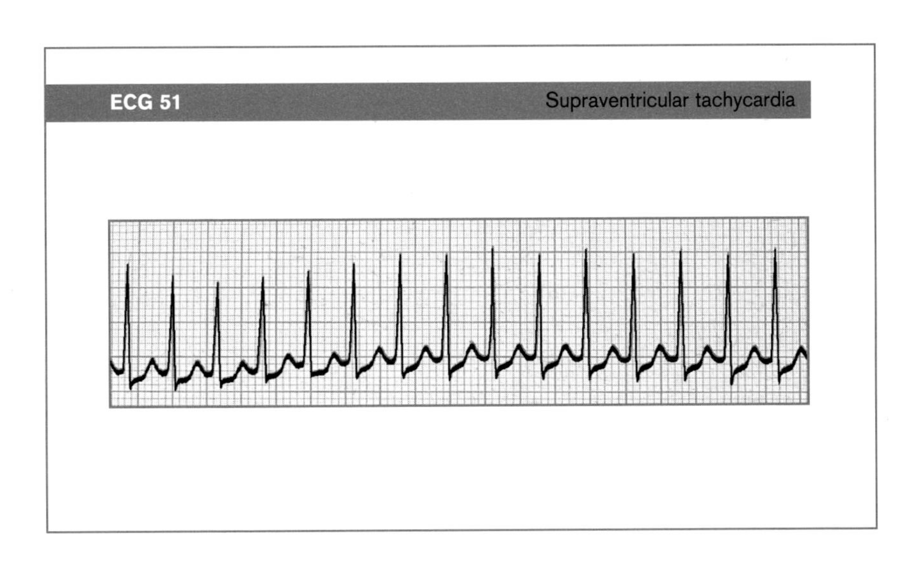

ECG 52-54: Broad complex tachycardias

Ventricular tachycardia

Ventricular ectopic rhythms arise when the focus that initiates ventricular depolarisation lies below the bifurcation of the bundle of His, either in the specialised conducting tissues or in the ventricular myocardium itself. At rates above 100 per minute ventricular tachycardia is present, while idioventricular rhythm is the term often used when the rate is slower. The QRS complex is broad, lasting more than 100 msec, reflecting the delayed activation of the ventricular myocardium that occurs under these circumstances.

Ventricular tachycardia is a dangerous arrhythmia; at fast rates or in the presence of impaired cardiac function, loss of cardiac output may result and cause cardiac arrest. It is also important to remember that ventricular tachycardia may precede the onset of ventricular fibrillation. Some examples of ventricular tachycardia are shown in **ECG 52-54**.

ECG 52: Ventricular tachycardia causing cardiac arrest. This is treated in the same way as ventricular fibrillation - by the application of electrical countershock.

ECG 52 Ventricular tachycardia

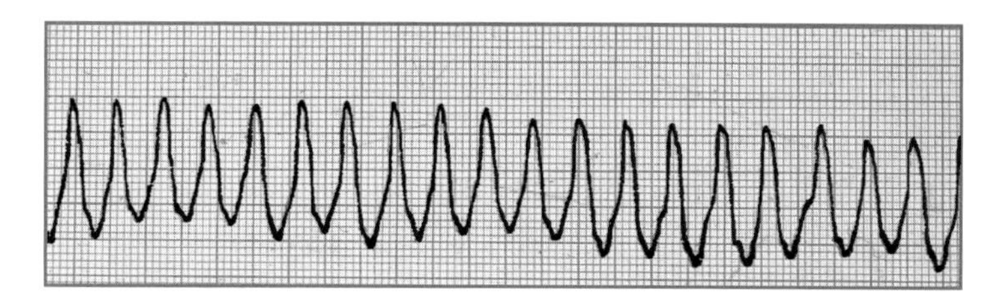

ECG 53 Ventricular tachycardia

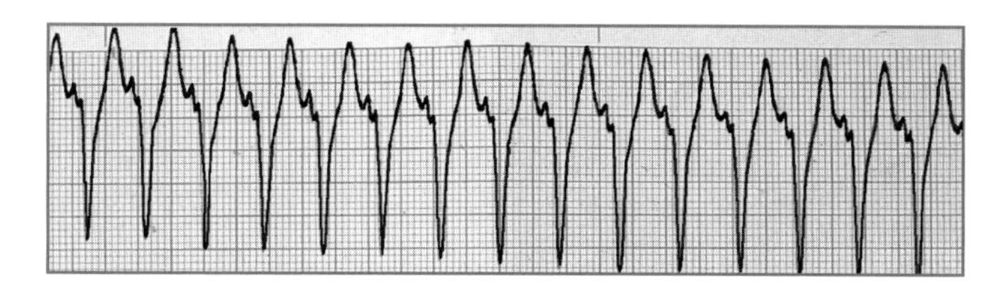

ECG 54 Ventricular tachycardia

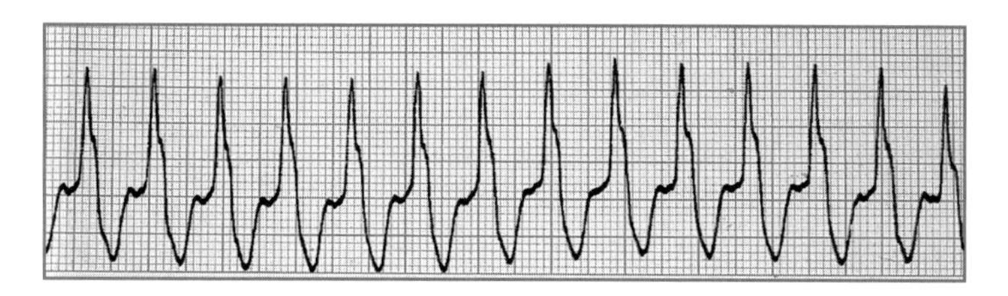

Aberrant conduction

A broad QRS complex tachycardia will also result when a rhythm arising above or within the AV junction is conducted aberrantly because right or left bundle branch block is present. In this situation it may be impossible to decide from a rhythm strip whether the rhythm is ventricular or supraventricular in origin, and a 12-lead ECG should be obtained in every case.

In the context of myocardial ischaemia the rhythm will nearly always be ventricular in origin, and the alternative diagnosis of a supraventricular tachycardia conducted aberrantly can usually be discounted.

ECG 55: Atrial fibrillation conduced aberrantly - note the basic irregularity of the rhythm.

ECG 56: Regular broad complex tachycardia. The 12-lead ECG - **ECG 57** helps to clarify the diagnosis as supraventricular tachycardia conducted with right bundle branch block.

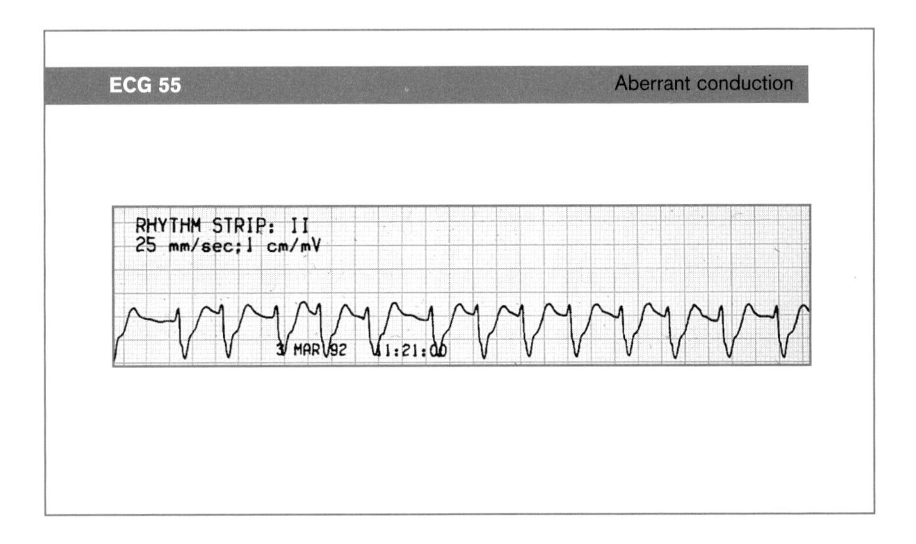

ECG 55 Aberrant conduction

ECG 56 Aberrant conduction

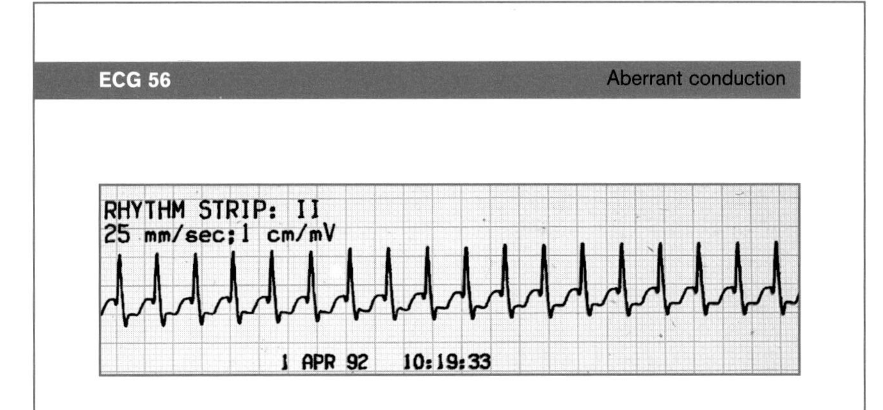

ECG 57 Aberrant conduction

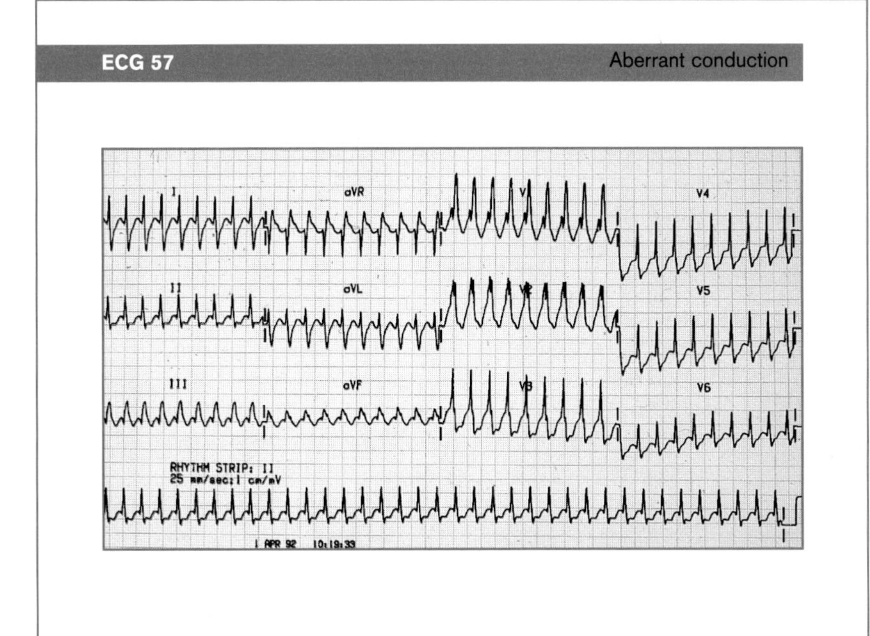

Q

R

S

T

U

V